Advance Praise for *Breath Taking*

"Astonishing...one of the most moving memoirs I've read. There is something to be learned from this book."
— CAROLINE LEAVITT, *New York Times* bestselling author of *Pictures of You* and *Days of Wonder*

"A tale of unimaginable loss imbued with humor, hope, and grace. *Breath Taking* captivated me from the very first sentence and left me glowing from the warmth of Jessica Fein's glorious appreciation for our imperfect world. This is not just a book; it's a master class in how to be a person."
— JOANNA RAKOFF, bestselling author of *My Salinger Year*

"A story of relentless heartbreak met with wit, strength, and resilience, Jessica Fein's memoir reminds us that optimism, perseverance, and ultimately acceptance are the keys to surviving life's curveballs. When the choices are curling up in the fetal position or facing adversity head-on, Fein has chosen the latter in spades. Her story is the perfect illustration of how we control nothing in life but our actions and attitude."
— JENNIFER WEISEL BAILEY, *ELLE* Magazine

"In *Breath Taking*, Jessica Fein finds the words to convey the deepest truths of being human and then shares them with vivid candor as if over a cup of coffee."
— RABBI SUSAN SILVERMAN, author of *Casting Lots: Creating a Family in a Beautiful, Broken World*

"This story truly matters and people need to hear it. *Breath Taking* is a remarkable celebration of resilience, and a true testament to strength, love, and survival. It shows us that there's always a path forward even when it's too dark to see. You'll probably laugh and cry, and you'll for sure be inspired."
—VICTORIA ARLEN, TV host, Paralympic gold medalist, and author

"Jessica throws aside pride and pretense expressing with generous vulnerability the heartbreaks and hopes that come with raising a child with a rare disease. More than an honest and humorous memoir, *Breath Taking* can be the guide star so many seek when life hands them more than they ever imagined they could endure."
—DANIEL DEFABIO, rare disease filmmaker and co-founder of the Disorder Channel

"Jessica Fein is that rare writer who can defuse sorrow with her sense of humor."
—DAN ZEVIN, Thurber Prize-winning humorist

"An epic story of love and resilience."
—KIRKLAND HAMILL, author of *Filthy Beasts*

"Jessica Fein puts a human face on the mystery of the rare disease world. Her memoir should be required reading for anyone entering the field."
—TERRI QUELER, MSW, LICSW, former associate professor of Genetic Counseling, Brandeis University

BREATH TAKING

A Memoir of Family, Dreams,
and Broken Genes

JESSICA FEIN

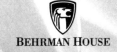

BEHRMAN HOUSE

NOTE FROM THE AUTHOR:
This is a work of nonfiction. Events and conversations are as
I remember them. Some names were changed to protect privacy and
some events were compressed. Any mistakes are my own.

Published by Behrman House, Inc.
Millburn, New Jersey 07041
www.behrmanhouse.com

ISBN 978-1-68115-110-6
ISBN (e-book) 978-1-68115-115-1

Library of Congress Cataloging-in-Publication Data

Names: Fein, Jessica, author.
Title: Breath taking : a memoir of family dreams and broken genes / Jessica Fein.
Description: Millburn, New Jersey : Behrman House, [2024] | Includes
bibliographical references. | Summary: "In 2010 Jessica Fein's adopted
daughter Dalia was diagnosed with a rare degenerative disease that would
ultimately claim her life. But before that moment came, Jessica and her
family would learn much about living with both hope and despair, loving
completely, accepting the unacceptable, and sharing not just strength,
but vulnerability and fear"-- Provided by publisher.
Identifiers: LCCN 2023035137 | ISBN 9781681151106 (hardcover)
Subjects: LCSH: Fein, Jessica--Family. | Parents of terminally ill
children--United States--Biography. | Epileptic children--United States.
| Mitochondrial DNA--Abnormalities.
Classification: LCC RJ249 .F45 2024 | DDC 618.92/8530092
[B]--dc23/eng/20230824
LC record available at https://lccn.loc.gov/2023035137

Edited by Aviva Lucas Gutnick
Jacket design by NeuStudio
Interior design by Zatar Creative

Flower image: BoxerX, Shutterstock

Printed in China

1 3 5 7 9 8 6 4 2

All around me,
the fireflies charge the world
with their beautiful, fleeting light.

ROSEMERRY WAHTOLA TROMMER

Contents

On March 11, 2022,
my daughter Dalia took her last breath.

But that's not what this story is about.

It's both the oldest story in the world,
and it's one you've never heard before.

This is a love story.

PART ONE

Mother May I?

1

Broken and Overflowing

When did I know something was wrong? People ask me this a lot. Depending on my mood, I answer one of two ways.

"I had a hunch from the start," I might say. "I always thought her ear looked funny. It was mottled and kind of squished. And the sounds she made were guttural. Aren't babies supposed to coo?"

Other times, I say, "We were shocked. We lived in ignorant bliss for nearly five years, completely mesmerized by our perfect little girl."

Both answers are true.

Our lives were fabulously chaotic, just like any family with working parents and three kids under seven. Desperate for time alone, one summer weekend my husband, Rob, and I hired a babysitter and drove an hour and a half to Newport, Rhode Island. We would have been just as excited to go to the Motel 6 across town. A weekend away meant we'd be able to talk, eat, and sleep together without little hands and big voices popping up between us.

Four hours in, my friend Lara called to check in. "We're having the best time," I told her. "The weather's perfect, and the hotel is fantastic. Even if it ended now, it will have been the best vacation ever."

Tempting the fates never worked out well for me.

Our vacation lasted seven hours. Seven glorious, uninterrupted, sunshiny hours.

We were settling into our chaises by the pool. "Is it too early to have a fruity drink?" I asked.

"We're on vacation. We can do whatever we want," Rob said, picking up the cocktail menu. Thirty seconds later, mid-sunscreen shmearing, my phone rang.

"Hi, it's Nicole," our four-year-old's teacher said in a rush, sounding scared. "Dalia fell and hit her head on the corner of a table. She has a huge gash near her eye. We called an ambulance, and we're on our way to the hospital."

I broke into a cold sweat as I watched the heat waves shimmering up off the patio around the pool. I started throwing my stuff into my beach bag.

"There's a lot of blood. I'm so sorry . . . I just turned my head for a second," Nicole said.

I put the phone on speaker, and Rob and I listened together as we hurried back to our room to grab our things.

"How's she doing?"

"She's being Dalia. The whole time we were waiting for the ambulance she kept patting my hand and saying, 'My okay, Miss Cole. Don't worry.'"

Getting phone calls that Dalia had fallen was nothing new, but this was the first time a fall was landing her in the hospital. As Rob ran to get the car, I wondered, for the hundredth-or-so time, whether I was massively failing at my primary maternal job of keeping my daughter safe.

At first, she'd met the standard milestones—rolling over, crawling, pulling up. But her toddling never matured into a steady gait. Instead she wobbled, as if tipsy, leaning on the wall to help steady herself. And her speech was garbled. She focused so intensely when she spoke. She looked like the effort thoroughly exhausted her, her tongue using every one of its eight muscles to propel the words out of her mouth.

But the doctor said she was fine. "Just give her more time," he told us. The team at Early Intervention said she didn't qualify for services. I convinced them to evaluate her three times, but the verdict never changed. "She's on the lower end of average," they said, and I felt bad that I was secretly hoping my daughter would rate below average and get help. I wondered if I was overreacting, if my expectations were too high. The worry gnawed at me.

Rob and I were quiet for the beginning of the car ride.

Finally I broke our silence. "What if she loses her eye?"

"Nicole would have told us if it was that bad," Rob said.

"You're right," I said, trying to mimic the deep breathing that made my yoga teacher look so relaxed.

A bit later it was Rob's turn.

"Why haven't we heard from Nicole? Let's call her again."

Rob and I had settled into the delicate dance that most parents know well. One worries, and the other reassures. Trade places; bow to your partner. We each knew when to advance and when to retreat. If we twirled together in the worry and fear, we would collapse.

But in my head, I didn't have to take turns. I could panic as much as I wanted. *It cannot be normal to fall as often as Dalia does. How many falls is it going to take for somebody to figure out what's going on?* I looked at the family in the car next to us. They look so calm, bored even. *Why can't we be like them? Haven't we had more than our fair share of pain? Why isn't Rob driving faster?*

Can we not even have one long weekend without any drama?

Rob pulled up to the hospital emergency room to drop me off. I opened the door before he stopped the car and ran inside. There was no line at the information desk, which was a good thing, because I would have knocked over anything that stood between me and my child.

"I'm looking for my daughter, Dalia Flaggert."

"Sure thing; let me see here," the receptionist said, tapping on her keyboard.

"Suze, I'm going to Dunkin' Donuts. Can I get you anything?" interrupted the valet guy at the next desk.

"Thanks, doll. I'll have a large latte with caramel drizzle and a splash of almond milk. Wait a second, let me get some money for you," she said, reaching for her purse.

Patience was not my strong suit under the best of circumstances, which these clearly weren't.

"Um, excuse me, Suze," I cut in. "I really need to find my daughter."

"Oh, sorry, honey," she said, turning back to her computer. "She's down the hall behind me in room three."

Rob came in just then. "Why are you still here? Where's Dalia?"

"Coffee," I said, taking his hand and heading down the hall. "Don't ask."

Dalia lay on a hospital bed cuddled with her teacher. There was a huge piece of gauze taped over one of her eyes, but when she saw us, her other eye lit up.

"Hi, Daddy. Hi, Mama," she smiled. Then came a frown: "My fell down." She held out her arms for a hug, and I felt like my heart was breaking and overflowing at the same time.

Later that night, after we'd clasped Dalia's hands while her eyelid was stitched up and held an ice pack on the egg on her forehead and explained to the boys why we were home from our vacation two days early and reassured them that Dalia was fine, that the stitches made it look worse than it was; after we told the babysitter she didn't need to stay, but yes of course we'd pay her anyway, and I crawled into bed, Rob brought me the drink I'd ordered at the pool.

"We'll go back to that hotel someday," he said. "It may not be for ten years, but we'll go back."

"Okay, but in the meantime, what about Dalia?" I asked, partly rhetorically and partly looking for the reassurance Rob was so good at.

"We're going to figure it out," he said. Because I wanted to believe him, and because I was exhausted, and because there was nothing more that could be done at that point in the night, I agreed.

2

Lightning Strikes

The path to becoming Dalia's mother was bumpy, full of more pivots and potholes than I could have imagined. In Judaism, the number eighteen means "life." So perhaps there's some spiritual symbolism that Dalia was placed in my arms for the first time on the eighteenth of September, exactly eighteen years from the first time I saw Rob, skateboarding across the University of Michigan campus.

What caught my eye was the ease with which he carried himself, the way so many people called out to him as he flew past in his Sonic Youth T-shirt. "Do you know that guy?" I asked my friend Shelly. She looked up from her book and took him in. "Not yet," she said.

I beat her to it and met Rob a few weeks later. On the surface, we were a textbook case of opposites attracting. Rob was a Midwesterner who'd grown up camping, trout fishing, and playing hockey. He was a Boy Scout but also into hard-core music and horror films. All three of those things scared me.

I was an East Coast urban Jew whose father taught me that the principal purpose of the human body was to keep one's head from rolling around on the ground. Ping-pong was my sport of choice. It was almost embarrassing when we watched *The Way We Were* together; Rob was so clearly the blue-eyed Robert Redford to my frizzy-haired Barbra Streisand.

Years earlier my mother told me to choose the person I had the most fun with. "Everything else comes and goes," she said, "looks, money, jobs, sex. If you're going to spend your life with someone, make sure it's somebody you just love to be with."

That was the bottom line with Rob. I just loved to be with him, and it wasn't only because he made me laugh harder than anyone I'd ever met. He knew things I didn't—what a sand dollar was and how to locate the Big Dipper, the difference between Parliament and Funkadelic, the etymology of the word "okay"—and he was curious about things I knew that he didn't. We balanced each other out—his patience to my urgency, his certainty about who he was to my eternal questioning, his comfort in solitude to mine in a crowd. He could focus on a single tree all day long, while I'd be racing to see the whole forest—a bit of a problem when we went hiking.

We dated through college and made our way to Seattle after graduation. Rob was drawn there by the rugged beauty and the throbbing music scene. I was drawn there by Rob.

But Seattle was rainy and way too far from family back in Boston. My sister Nomi, three years older and my best friend, was pregnant, and living in different time zones wasn't going to work for us when she became a mother.

I was the second person Nomi told when she found out she was pregnant. I'd just arrived from Seattle for Passover when Nomi pulled me up the stairs and into my old bedroom.

"Do I look different?" she asked. I looked her up and down. Long, thick, curly hair—same as always; same as mine.

Big green eyes and impossibly perfect body, which was particularly annoying given her undisciplined diet that included a daily Hershey's bar and her tendency to eat a full can of black olives in one sitting. "No, you look exactly the same," I said, completing my assessment.

"Look again," she said, sticking out her washboard stomach. I looked at her stomach and then looked up at her face. I noticed her big eyes were open even wider than usual, and her smile was unfamiliar.

I knew my sister's smiles. There was the performance smile she'd mastered for the variety show our older sister, Rachel, directed us in for years. Nomi was the Golde to my Tevye, the Peaches to my Herb. We never actually performed the show in front of an audience, but we practiced dutifully should the opportunity ever arise.

There was the smile when she wanted me to do something for her, like literally give her the shirt off my back because she thought my outfit was cuter than hers. There was the smile of encouragement that telepathically said, "You've got this, and what's more, I've got you," like when she showed up at my high school orientation to help me navigate from one class to the next or when she helped me hide my hangover from our mother the first time I got drunk.

There was the "I'm smarter than you smile," which she pulled out sparingly, which was generous since she actually was smarter.

And there was the truly, deeply happy smile, like when she introduced me to David, the man she'd end up marrying.

But this was a new smile—one I hadn't seen before.

"Oh my God, you're pregnant," I screamed.

She nodded, and I hugged her tightly—but not too tightly —around her stomach. I quickly scanned my bookshelf for my old copy of *Our Bodies, Ourselves.* "Okay, the baby is the size of a sweet pea," I said, flipping through the pages. "How big is a sweet pea? What exactly is a sweet pea, and how is it different from a regular pea? Wait! How are you gonna tell David?"

She looked at me, eyebrows slightly raised. "Right, you've already told David," I realized.

Once we moved to Boston, my family swirled around us. Rob and I lived in an apartment just a five-minute walk from my childhood home, where my mother and stepfather, Frank, still lived.

My ninety-five-year-old grandmother, Bub, lived right across the street from us in a senior housing complex. "It makes me feel young to have you so close," she told me. "Everybody here treats me like I'm one hundred."

The proximity to my family felt a bit shtetl-like, equal parts suffocating and comforting. Growing up with divorced parents, I was used to splitting the holidays. Now, Rob and I often split the weekends—Friday night dinner with one parent, Sunday brunch with the other. Meals with my mom followed a formula: over-dressed salad, sloppy chicken, and rice pilaf, followed by all of us gathering around the piano, where we sang along while my mom played from her *Jewish Songs Old and New* piano book. The first time Rob observed this particular ritual, I worried he might board the next plane back to Seattle. But the second time, he found Frank watching the Red Sox in the den and joined him there. Frank silently handed Rob a beer, and a beautiful friendship was formed.

Meals with my dad were less predictable, as the topics of conversation moved quickly from the crisis in Ethiopia to my father's plan to solve world hunger to rapid exchanges of wildly inappropriate jokes, which my father always told in a feigned Yiddish accent, even if the joke took place in Sweden. Every story my father told started the same way, "It happened in Minsk, or maybe it was Pinsk." We never found out which.

Somehow Rob fit right in. His intellectual curiosity appealed to my father. His sense of humor, ability to fix things, and good looks charmed my mother. He quickly became Bub's favorite. She put on lipstick when she saw him come through the door and stopped the rest of us from eating our first piece of cake lest Rob want a second. "Leave it for the boyfriend!" she commanded in her thick Russian accent.

Life wasn't perfect, but it was close. My mid-level marketing job paid my half of the rent and allowed for a bit of creativity. Rob was working during the day and was in graduate school at night, so I had lots of time to get my family fix with Nomi and my brand-new niece, Liat.

This was my age of innocence.

—»·«—

One stormy January day, Nomi called me at work to debrief about the weekend wedding she had attended and to ask for a book recommendation. By then Nomi was a stay-at-home mom. She called me every day when Liat was napping, oblivious to the fact that I had a job and that talking to her wasn't part of it.

A few hours later, my father called for the second time that day. We'd already had our daily morning chat. "What, Dad?" I asked, annoyed nobody in my family understood that taking personal calls from my cubicle was not the strategy to get me out of my mid-level job and into a private office.

"Nomi collapsed," he blurted.

"What are you talking about?" I asked, my face starting to burn. "I just spoke to her. She's fine."

"David called and said she collapsed while playing with Liat. They took her to the hospital in an ambulance. That's all I know. Just grab your stuff and meet me out front."

It took us forty-five minutes to get to the hospital. Over and over we told ourselves that Nomi had simply fainted. We weren't even sufficiently concerned to pick up Rachel or my mother on the way.

We checked in at the emergency room reception and were escorted into a private meeting room, where David was sobbing and shaking his head. The doctor told us Nomi had gone into sudden cardiac arrest and died instantly. He needn't have said a thing. As soon as I saw David, I knew Nomi was gone.

One by one, family and friends materialized at the hospital. I have no idea who called them to share the news. But I couldn't reach Rob, who was in class. I sat in a chair in the corner of the room shaking. I didn't sob or reach for a hug or use the hospital phone to make calls. I just shook. I wasn't the least bit cold, but I was shivering from my scalp to my toes.

At some point someone drove me back to Nomi and David's house, where people started to congregate. I don't remember who drove me. I don't know whether we were at the hospital for thirty minutes or three hours. All I remember is the shaking.

In college, my roommate Kim had an old Toyota that would shake at speeds above fifty miles per hour. Driving on the highway always felt like being on a rickety carnival ride. We used to joke that at some point the car would simply shake itself apart. My body's response to Nomi's sudden death didn't feel like being in that car; it felt like I was that car. I was certain that at any minute I'd fall apart.

A friend of my mother's pulled me aside and said, "You need to take care of your mother now. Losing a child is the worst thing that can happen to anybody." How she thought I was in any condition to take care of my mother was beyond me. Wasn't my mother going to be taking care of me? Well-meaning people brought me bagels and cups of water and glasses of wine. I wanted none of it.

The house got crowded as word spread. I recognized several people from Nomi's thirtieth birthday parties a few months earlier. There had been three separate celebrations to mark the occasion. She had too many friends to squeeze into just one.

Finally, Rob arrived. He wrapped me in his arms, and I stopped shaking and started to cry.

– ›› ‹‹ –

Nomi's death poked a massive hole in the bubble I'd lived in up to that point. I tried to patch it up, but it was no use. There would be many more losses to come, each one shaped by that first one. I started to see the world not through the hazy sheen of my bubble, but through the clarity of the puncture.

Back then, I said there was no way I could go on without my sister. I said, "It makes no sense" and "It's not fair" and "This wasn't our plan." If that conversation took place with the me of today, I'd laugh in that naïve young woman's face (not in a rude way, of course, she being me and all). Because everything that's happened to me since has proved over and over that any notion of fairness or order is a fantasy; that there's painful truth in the Yiddish proverb printed on the mug my cousin Karen gave me, "Man plans, and God laughs."

But I didn't know any of that then. What I did know, though, is that Rob and I would marry soon after and spend the rest of our lives together, not only because he was my favorite person, but also because I knew he could stop my shaking in a storm.

We had a lot to mourn the night we got married but also a lot to celebrate. The sadness and the joy danced together, each perhaps more powerful because of the other.

3

Try and Try Again

Within a year I threw away my diaphragm. On vacation, in a basement apartment in my cousins' home in Jerusalem, we had unprotected sex for the first time.

The next morning, I was struck with the certainty that I was pregnant, that my body was busy knitting together our first child, a future concert violinist or vascular surgeon. My theoretical pregnancy put a damper on the rest of our travels through Israel and Italy, as I didn't want to push myself too hard given my expectant state. I walked gingerly up Mount Masada, making the already long ascent take twice as long, and I never sampled the wines at the Tuscan vineyards we drove hours to find.

When I got my period on the plane ride home, I wasn't merely disappointed but genuinely surprised. I chalked the failure up to international travel and assumed we'd have success four weeks later.

That surprise disappointment repeated itself every month for the next year.

It was a blessing and a curse that my sister Rachel was also having trouble getting pregnant. I could confide in her that for a second I thought about ramming my grocery cart into the pregnant woman at Stop & Shop whose T-shirt read, "Baby on Board," and she'd know exactly what I meant. She could describe her spotting, and together we'd try to decipher whether it was a sign of implantation or her period. But the fact that the person we most wanted to get pregnant other than ourselves was also failing nearly doubled our disappointment each month.

Rachel was eight years older, and for most of our lives I'd thought of her as a slightly mysterious, glamorous template for who I might become when I grew up. When I was five, she sat Nomi and me down, pulled out the book *Where Did I Come From?* and explained in graphic detail how babies were made. When I was eight, I parked myself on the stairs and watched when Richie Greenberg came to pick her up for her first date. I stayed on the stairs until she returned three hours later to see whether they kissed on our front porch. When I was twelve, Nomi and I visited Rachel at college in Chicago. She showed us off at the library and took us to a football game and introduced us to deep-dish pizza. When the three of us curled up in Rachel's twin bed that night, Nomi and I decided that when the time came, we'd both go to college there too.

But now the chasm between us narrowed. We were peers in our pursuit of motherhood. If we were going to sit on the sidelines and watch everyone else parade by with pregnant bellies and toddlers in tow, at least we could sit there together, sharing a blanket and passing hot chocolate back and forth.

Because now all my friends were having babies. One by one I got the phone call, mustered up a passable degree of enthusiasm, went to the baby shower, came home, and cried.

Every day seemed like "Baby Day!" at Target and Stop & Shop and even at the gym. No matter where I was, I saw pregnant women holding their hands protectively over their bellies as though they were carrying a particularly delicate Jell-O mold. They looked so full, and I felt so empty.

Adding insult to emotional injury, I worked for a childcare company and spent hours a day writing marketing copy to appeal to pregnant moms and selecting photos of babies for brochures. I studied the pictures of the parents holding their newborn prizes. *Why them and not me?*

And so when we were thirty-one, Rob and I entered a throuple with the Boston medical community. We started with a relatively simple procedure, intrauterine insemination, in which the doctor inserted Rob's sperm into my uterus during ovulation. It was like giving the sperm a way to skip a stormy rush-hour traffic jam and be delivered gingerly to the perfect parking spot at their final destination.

It seemed like we were outsmarting Intro to Biology with an advanced placement course. How could it not work?

But month after month, the missing plus sign taunted us.

Rachel and her husband had moved on to in vitro fertilization, and she persuaded me to call her doctor. "Maybe they'll give us a two-for-one deal."

Now we were growing whole embryos to put in my uterus. As long as I could provide a hospitable environment for them, we'd be all set.

No exercise, no wine, no stress (ha!).

And, as it turned out, no pregnancy.

Was it possible that my stress about not getting pregnant was keeping me from getting pregnant? I signed up for a mind-body class for women struggling with infertility.

The instructor spoke in a hypnotic voice as she taught us how to breathe. "Breathe in through your nose for four counts, breathe out for six. Pick a mantra to repeat while you're breathing. Try 'hmmmmmmm' when you breathe in," she suggested, "'saaaaaaaaa' when you breathe out. Hmmmmmmm . . . saaaaaaaaa."

It sounded so peaceful when she said it, so relaxing. Later that night I woke up in a cold sweat, my mind racing. *My stomach hurts. Is that a good sign or a bad sign? Is it too early for morning sickness, and can it happen in the middle of the night? Why did I eat the second bowl of frozen yogurt? Hmm-saa, Hmm-saa, Hmm-saa.*

It didn't work. I got out of bed and ate another bowl of frozen yogurt.

— ›› ‹‹ —

"There is another option," the doctor said after a third year went by. "Since your embryos are strong, you could use a gestational carrier, someone with a track record of successful pregnancy."

It sounded kind of awesome.

"What do you think?" I asked Rob, as we got into our car.

"I think it's totally bizarre," he said.

This wasn't the resounding enthusiasm I'd hoped for. "Totally bizarre in a good way, though, right?"

"We'd be essentially renting space in somebody else's body. How can we trust a complete stranger? It feels really risky. I need some time to think about it."

"Have you thought about it?" I asked as we walked into our house, annoying even myself.

It took him a full day, but Rob agreed to give it a go, and within a couple of months, we signed a contract with Christine, a Midwesterner who was joining the ever-expanding cast of characters in our baby-making pursuit.

When it came time for Christine to come to Boston for the embryo transfer, she told me she'd be bringing her husband, Steve, along for the adventure and that they'd feel most connected to us if they stayed in our home. Frankly, that was a bit more connection than we were looking for. We preferred to think of Christine's uterus as somewhat separate from Christine—a substitution for my uterus, not a substitution for me. And honestly, who was Steve in this whole operation anyway?

But if everything worked as we were hoping and paying for, they'd be giving our baby a home for nine months. It felt a bit selfish to say no to hosting them for a couple of days.

They were scheduled to arrive at 5:00 p.m. I asked my mother to get there by 2:00 to cook a dinner I could pretend I'd made. I wanted Christine to see how domestic I was—to think I was bursting with maternal prowess. And I needed my parents to be there with us to offset the strangers in the room with the people closest to me.

I had pregame conversations with each of them.

"Do not bring up politics or religion," I instructed my mother.

Mom was a fiery, indomitable, intense intellectual. She guzzled screwdrivers and laughed easily and said "Shit on a goddamn fucking stick" when she was frustrated. Her name was Zelda, and she was everything you might imagine someone named Zelda would be. Her huge personality burst out of her five-foot, two-inch frame. She was the exclamation point at the end of the alphabet, overflowing with vim and vigor. Never mind the fact that embarrassed by her name, she preferred to be called "Bonnie" in public; she was "Zelda" through and through. I adored everything about her. I just didn't want "everything" to be on display on this particular occasion.

"What are you so worried about?" my father asked when I told him which topics were off the table.

"What I'm worried about is that you'll talk about politics just like you did when you met Rob's parents, even though I begged you not to."

My father started his career as a political science professor at MIT and was now a writer and speaker about politics in general and American Jews in particular. Asking him not to talk about religion or politics at a dinner party was like inviting Baryshnikov to the stage and asking him not to dance.

Neither of my parents was comfortable taking the back seat conversationally, but it was their solid presence I needed that night, not their big personalities.

All went smoothly on the conversational front at first. But somewhere between the salad and the sloppy chicken, we started talking about Christine and Steve's drive to Boston.

"It would have been better if we could have driven around New York instead of through it," Christine started. "The traffic was crazy."

"Everything about New York is a mess," Steve chimed in. "And it doesn't help that Hillary Clinton is now their senator. Honestly, I'd be happy if I never hear her name again."

Shit, I thought.

I looked at my mother across the table, beseeching her with my eyes not to engage. I saw her biting her cheek, trying not to defend Hillary, not to share that I recently gave her the new Hillary Clinton coffee-table book for Hanukkah.

Hold it in, Mom, I said to her without talking. *Are you kidding me?* she replied silently. *How can you expect me to be quiet when they're insulting Hillary?*

Do it for me, Mom, my eyes replied. *I need this to go well. I need them to like us.*

Our silent conversation about Hillary was interrupted when Christine dug into her purse and pulled out a small jewelry box. "I was going to wait until tomorrow to give this to you, but now seems like as good a time as any." She awkwardly reached across the table and handed it to me. I wondered for a split second if the fact that she was going to carry a baby for me meant she thought she ought to propose to me too.

I opened the box and pulled out a gold necklace with a pendant of a mother holding her baby. It was very convincing. *I'm going to be a mother. I might be getting there in a round-about way, but it's going to happen. I will be just as much of a mom as all those pregnant women in Target and Stop & Shop.*

The next morning, proudly wearing the necklace, I trooped to the hospital with Rob, Christine, and Steve for the embryo transfer. I held Christine's hand and watched the doctor insert two healthy embryos into her uterus.

Two weeks later the test came back negative.

I called Christine. She started sobbing, and I consoled her. My loss, her tears, my sympathy.

"It's okay. I know you did everything you could. It wasn't meant to be," I said. But really what I was saying was, *"Are you kidding me? We can't even get somebody else pregnant? But I was wearing the necklace!"*

I was so tired of mustering up hope and feeling like a crashing failure. We'd already come to terms with the fact that I wasn't going to carry our baby. Was it really that important that she be ours biologically? Maybe not.

I decided to broach the subject gently with Rob, putting together an exhaustive list of the benefits of moving to adoption.

"Sweetie, I'm tired," I began.

"I know you're tired. It's 8:00 and we're in bed."

"No, I'm *tired*," I tried again. "I'm tired of all of it. I'm tired of trying so hard. I'm tired of feeling so bad. I think maybe we should start considering adoption. I've been thinking . . ."

"Yeah, I think so too," Rob said, before I could even get to the first item on my twelve-point list.

"But wait! I have a list!" I said. "Don't you want to hear the list?"

"I'd love to hear your list. But let's do it."

I made a spreadsheet with variables about each country, weighing things like how old the babies typically were when adoptions were finalized, length of the process from start to finish, and whether the babies were in orphanages or foster care. We went to "information nights," where we sipped soda from plastic cups and ate sugar cookies while we walked around the room studying posters of children born in a dozen countries we knew little about.

Guatemala soon emerged as the place with the most pluses in our country scorecard.

We became newly energized by what we no longer thought of as baby-making, but as family-building. The illusion that we had some control here was powerful. Never mind that we were preparing to intertwine ourselves for eternity with someone born in another part of the world to a woman we were unlikely ever to meet. We felt, at last, like we were in charge.

I even began parking in the "expectant mother" parking space at the mall nearby, hoping someone would have the gall to challenge my claim to the spot.

One night, Rob and I got a bottle of wine, ordered Chinese food, and dug into the ream of adoption paperwork.

The first set of questions asked what medical conditions we'd "be open to." There were check-off boxes next to medical conditions we'd heard of and a few we hadn't. "HIV, blindness, deafness . . ."–the list went on and on. We looked at each other. I didn't want to answer first. What if we didn't see eye to eye? Would Rob think less of me when I told him I didn't want a baby with extra needs?

After a minute, Rob started. "I'm fine with any of these . . . truly. I've always thought I'd be good with a special-needs child. Some cultures think those kids are closer to God."

Oh shit. I didn't even think Rob believed in God, and now I had to confess that he was a better person than I was. I took a gulp of wine. "I don't know . . . I just don't think I want that." I studied the chicken and broccoli on my plate for a minute before looking up. "Is that horrible?"

"No, maybe you're right," he said, taking a bite of moo shu. "It would probably be overwhelming. What's the next question?"

"Please share why you wish to adopt a child."

It felt like a test, and I was afraid we were going to fail.

"How about we say, 'We're eager to extend the love and respect we have for each other to a child, whom we'll welcome into our home with all the joy every baby deserves,'" Rob offered. "Yes!" I said, leaning awkwardly across the table to kiss him.

Rob stated it formally, very English-teacher-like. But he was right. We had obscene amounts of love to give, and we never looked at adopting as a consolation prize. It wasn't that we came to terms with adopting; we became committed to it. We felt powerfully connected to the parentless children whose pictures we'd seen, because we felt like we were childless parents. We suspected that there was a child or two in Guatemala who were supposed to be ours, and it was just a matter of time before they came home to us.

4

Finally Family

Guatemala is a Central American country tucked in between Mexico, Honduras, Belize, El Salvador, and the Pacific Ocean. It's the most highly populated country in Central America by far, but just the third largest in terms of area—slightly larger than Tennessee. The official language is Spanish, though more than twenty distinct Mayan languages are spoken there. About half the labor force works in agriculture, and more than half the population lives below the national poverty level. The Guatemalan Civil War lasted from 1960 to 1996, killing about two hundred thousand people. We have Guatemala to thank for chocolate and what many consider the world's best coffee.

But I didn't know any of that when we traveled there for the first time. I'm mortified to admit I couldn't find Guatemala on a map, yet I knew it would be the place where my life would change forever.

One night, what felt like an eternity after we'd completed the adoption paperwork, our social worker from Wide Horizons, Jane, called us. "I have good news. Are you sitting down? Is Rob there? You might want to put me on speaker."

"There's a nine-month-old boy who's ready to be adopted. He's with a foster mother in Guatemala City. I'm looking at his picture right now. I'll be emailing it over to you in a minute."

"Oh my God, oh my God, oh my God," was all I could say. A nine-month-old boy. Ready for us. Our child.

"What happens now? When can we go? What should we do?" We pummeled Jane with questions.

We could hear her smile. "For now, I just want you to look at the information I'm sending you. It'll be about three months before we'll get a court date, so we have time. Oh, and it would be a good idea to start carrying around a twenty-pound bag of rice."

I thanked her and hung up. As I raced to get the computer, Rob asked, "Did she just tell us to start carrying rice?" "I don't know," I called from the other room, before I rushed back in, logging onto the computer.

And there he was. Looking right at us with big, brown, sparkling eyes, wearing a tiny white cardigan. We looked at the picture for hours that night and every day after. If everything worked out, this was the little person who would miraculously turn us into parents. We studied him, trying to interpret every clue. It looks like a hot day; why is he wearing a sweater? Is one of his pupils slightly off-center? Whose arm is that in the picture? Seems like another child's. And . . . He looks happy, right? He looks smart, right? He looks kind, right?

I printed that picture and carried it with me everywhere, feeling more of a claim to him each day. And we began waiting again. Now we were waiting for a specific person, not just the idea of a person.

We decided not to put the nursery together until we were assigned a court date. We were just too nervous this would fail. We bought small presents—toys and stuffed animals—and sent them to Guatemala. We slept with the stuffed animals before we sent them so our smell would become recognizable to our baby.

Three months went by, and we still didn't have a court date. Our baby was having his first birthday and we were missing it. "He's getting older," we told Jane. "He needs us." But what we meant was, "We need him." Another month passed, and then another. We kept the door to the room that would become the nursery closed.

In May, Rachel and her husband adopted a newborn from New Hampshire. When he was a week old, we celebrated his *bris*, which is when the Jewish community comes together for a baby's circumcision. Rachel gave me the honor of carrying her infant into the room and handing him to the rabbi. My parents beamed. Rachel beamed. I tried to beam, but in the pictures it looked like I'd just taken a bite out of a lemon.

After the ceremony, I snuck into Rachel's bedroom and called Jane. "No adoptions have moved through the system," she said. "I'll call you as soon as I hear anything."

I called Jane weekly, asking for updates, begging for good news. "Soon," she promised.

We went to Rob's family's cottage in Canada, a trip we'd hoped to miss. To be fair, I hoped to miss that trip every year. The cottage was exactly in the middle of nowhere. The only thing to do there was fish or relax, and I wasn't a fan of either. But that year the quiet and tranquility of the cottage were almost too much to bear. There was too much time to think about the grandchild I hadn't yet produced. The toys Rob and his brothers played with as kids were piled neatly on shelves in the guestroom, waiting to be brought back to life. The bunkbeds remained unmade.

Then one day, Jane called me at work. "Your case has been cleared," she said. "Your court date is next week. Buy your plane tickets."

We had a week to get ready for our twenty-two-pound, fifteen-month-old baby. We needed to be briefed and plan for what would happen when we got to Guatemala. We needed a stroller, a car seat, a high chair, and a crib. We had to put the nursery together and babyproof our home.

Maybe it's not surprising after all that I didn't have time to figure out where exactly Guatemala is located.

– ❯❯ ❮❮ –

The thing I remember most vividly about that first trip to Guatemala isn't meeting our son for the first time or signing the papers that bound us to him or marveling at his tininess as he napped on Rob's chest. All those moments are permanently etched in my heart, but the thing that sticks in my mind more than anything else is the elevator ride from the sixth floor down to the lobby of the Marriott on the morning of August 18, 2003.

We'd gotten the call a few minutes earlier, telling us that our group was waiting for us in the lobby. "Okay, they're here," I said to Rob in a trembling voice neither of us recognized. He took my hand, and we headed to the elevator.

We had six stories until we officially became parents, and it was both the longest and shortest ride of my life. We traveled five years to get to this elevator, to be in this exact spot at this exact time. It felt like the world's lengthiest gestational period—a mockery of the year-and-a-half record previously held by elephant mamas.

When we stepped into the lobby, we spotted Jonah, in his little white cardigan, right away. The foster mother greeted me with a hug and placed Jonah in my arms, and I was both in my body and outside of it. Here was Jonah, the sweetest, handsomest, mine-est child I'd ever seen. "Hi, sweetie, hi, hi," I kept repeating, trying to fast-forward my introduction to him and his to me. And yet there was a piece of me that felt self-conscious, as if we were on display for the foster mother and the rest of the group. I still felt like we had something to prove, that we had to convince them we were parental enough for them to leave this child with us.

And I wasn't entirely convinced myself.

We all returned to our room on the sixth floor. When Jonah started squirming in my lap, I looked to the foster mom.

She looked at me and said, "Esta bien, puedes dejarlo. Estara bien." Oscar translated, "It's okay, you can put him down. He'll be fine."

I followed behind, worried that he'd try to climb out the window or flush himself down the toilet, while Rob took diligent notes on Jonah's schedule, diet, and sleep habits. An hour passed and it was time for goodbyes.

The foster mother picked up Jonah. She whispered to him in Spanish. She hugged him. And then she made the sign of the cross on his tiny forehead, his little chest. It was so loving, so protective. I almost asked her to do it to me, too, but figured it likely wouldn't take given my Jewishness.

And then they were gone, and it was our first night as a family. We curled up on the hotel bed. Rob held Jonah on his stomach, and I rubbed our little son's back. "Hi, sweetie," I said softly, over and over. And then Jonah looked at me, smiled, and said, "Hi." But what I heard was so much more: "Hi, Mama. Here I am. I know you've been waiting for me for five years and for your whole life, and I've been waiting for you too. Let's be a family."

5

Always I Love Her Very Much

We were on a family-building roll.

We found out about Dalia, who at the time was named Daniela, when she was two weeks old. I was at work when her photo came through my email.

I grabbed my laptop and ran into my friend Ilene's office.

"She's here! She's so new. I mean, I must say she's not exactly the cutest baby I've ever seen. Her ear looks kind of squished, don't you think? And she seems to have kind of a furry forehead."

"Yes, but check out her hair," Ilene said. "It's incredible."

She was right. Dalia had a full head of thick black hair, even as a newborn. It was like she came out wearing a fur hat.

A few months later we flew to Guatemala to meet our baby girl. By now we knew the ropes, and we arrived with a bit of a been-there-done-that swagger. But as soon as I called our translator Oscar, our confidence dissolved.

"It's so good to speak to you," Oscar said, when I told him we'd arrived. "We'll meet you at the hotel in two hours. Do you have a large enough room? I'm bringing the foster mother and your baby, and also the baby's mother and grandmother."

"I'm sorry, what?" I asked, not fully comprehending the cast of characters that was accompanying him.

"We're on our way," he repeated, even though that wasn't the part I was confused about. "Wait for us in the lobby."

Oscar called Daniela/Dalia "your baby." There was an actual baby with Oscar at that very minute who was going to be mine. *A baby. But how could she also be with her mother and grandmother? Was she theirs too?*

Years before, when I made a spreadsheet to compare what I thought of as the "pluses" and "minuses" of different country's adoption policies, I put an X by Guatemala in the column that said, "Will we meet the birth parents?" On balance, that seemed like a positive. As adoptive parents, we were beholden to the birth parents. We knew they were heroes—people brave enough to admit that for whatever reason they weren't able to take care of a child—generous enough to give us that job.

But that didn't mean we actually wanted to meet them. Meeting them was a bit more real than we were prepared for. Meeting them forced us to belie the fantasy that our children spontaneously appeared out of a magical bubble, like Glinda the Good Witch.

While we understood that objectively this was an important and unusual opportunity, a chance to learn a bit more about Dalia's story, to put a face to her history and gather information we could share with her later, subjectively we were completely freaking out.

What if the mother and grandmother changed their minds when they saw the baby they'd put in foster care just three months earlier? What if they didn't like us and decided to wait for another couple? How could we claim this child as our own when the person who gave birth to her was sitting right there?

We found two strategically located seats in the lobby, where we could see people entering before they could see us. I studied each baby girl who was carried in to see if there was any resemblance to the picture I held.

After about twenty minutes, a woman entered the lobby carrying a tiny girl in an adorable lavender romper.

"I think it's her," I said, grabbing Rob's arm.

He studied the baby for a minute. "I'm not sure."

"Yes, look at her eyes, look at her ear." I took a little gasp, held my breath, and popped out of my chair in one motion. I walked across the lobby, detouring around large potted trees and wicker chairs, over to the foster mother, all the while gazing at the gorgeous baby. When I was just about there, I was cut off by another woman wearing the same dazzled expression I was. She reached out to embrace the girl, who was, it turned out, her daughter, not mine.

Rob just shook his head when I returned to my seat.

"Well, I guess that wasn't my proudest parenting moment," I said. "I just mistook a complete stranger for my daughter." It was the first time I said "my daughter" out loud. It was worth the mistake.

Almost an hour later a group of three women and a baby entered the lobby. This was Dalia. I knew her right away by that incredible head of hair. She was with a beautiful young woman with waves of black hair, who we'd find out was her birth mother, Ana; her grandmother, who looked our age; and the foster mother, who was holding Dalia. As Oscar introduced us, the foster mother handed Dalia to me.

I held her delicately and a bit clumsily. She was so tiny. I didn't introduce myself, being careful not to say, "I'm your mama," as I had with Jonah. The relationships here were too confusing. Instead, I quietly narrated as we walked, "We're going to go see our room, sweet girl, okay? Let's go for a ride in the elevator." I hoped my tone conveyed the absolute wonder I felt.

Had I had time to envision this meeting, I would have imagined that most of the conversation would be between the birth mother and Rob and me, that she would be driving the discussion and we'd feel deferential to her. But it was the foster mother's show. She was the one who told us all about our shared baby girl, how she giggled at silly faces and liked to have her forehead stroked as she was falling asleep. Everyone else in the room was riveted by her words. This was the last thing the birth mother and grandmother would likely know about Daniela, the first Rob and I were learning about Dalia.

As they were getting ready to leave, Oscar asked if we had any final questions for Ana.

"Have you had any other children?" I asked, and Oscar translated.

"No, this is the only one, and I won't have another."

I didn't put much stock in her answer. She seemed too young to be that sure of anything.

"Is there anything we can tell Dalia about you when she gets older?" asked Rob.

She smiled a little and touched Dalia's, her Daniela's, head gently. "Sempra te seguiré amando."

"Always I love her very much," Oscar translated.

Rob wrote her message down in a tiny notebook. They were just six English words, but he wanted to get them exactly right when he shared them with Dalia in the future.

"One more thing," Oscar said as they were walking out. "You'll need to get special formula for the baby. She has a sensitive stomach and can only tolerate this kind," he said, handing us an empty can. "I wish I could take you myself, but I have to drive everyone back home, which is going to take several hours. I suggest you walk to one of the *farmacias* in the neighborhood and see if you can find more there."

Rob set out on a quest for special formula, which sounds a bit Indiana Jones-ish and isn't unlike how he felt. I don't know which one of us was more nervous—him, as he wandered the neighborhood we'd been told by the adoption agency not to explore, or me, who was now alone in the hotel room with a three-month-old.

I'd never taken care of such a new human being before, and I was confident I'd figure out how to completely screw up. I was petrified that something would happen to Dalia in the first few minutes of my watch. So I did the most maternal thing I could think of: I called my mother back in Boston and asked her to stay on the phone with me until Rob got back. My mother was more than happy to oblige. I held the phone to Dalia's ear so she could hear Zelda serenade her with Yiddish lullabies. I don't know what Dalia thought of them, but they calmed me right down.

Rob returned about an hour later.

"I needed to go to three different *farmacias* to find the right formula," he said, passing me the plastic bag he was carrying. "The shopkeeper at the first one said it didn't matter what kind I bought. He kept trying to show me the ingredients were the same, but I didn't want to risk it. The next one didn't even carry formula. And I kept passing the same McDonalds, so I definitely think I was lost. How's she doing?" he asked, reaching out to scoop Dalia off the bed.

"I kept her safe for a full hour," I boasted.

I'm not sure which of us was prouder of our accomplishment.

The next day, feeling newly emboldened by our success on day one, we decided to venture out from our hotel.

We were experts at baby equipment now, so it took just a couple of minutes to attach the baby carrier to my body, situate Dalia safely in the harness, and cover her with a loose-knit poncho before we headed out.

"We're going outside for a walk," I whispered to Dalia, rubbing her back. This was the closest I ever got to the feeling I imagine newly pregnant women have. I felt like my whole world was different. I was protecting a treasure no one could see, yet it completely overpowered everything about me. I knew I was glowing.

— ❯❯ ❮❮ —

Three months later I still felt like I was glowing. We were home on an ordinary March evening, bathing Jonah and Dalia. I was singing one of my favorites.

"Manamana bum bum baddada. Manamana, bum badda bum..." I was singing and splashing, and the kids were giggling. But Rob was quiet.

"What's going on?" I asked, looking at his reflection in the mirror.

"If we don't get another baby, I think I'll always feel like somebody is missing."

I didn't want to be responsible for Rob spending his whole life thinking somebody was missing. Also, he chose a perfect time to make his case. There was nothing cuter than seeing those two babies in a bathtub full of bubbles. One more? More bubbles. More cuteness. Bring it on.

6

Family Tree

A few months after bringing Dalia home from Guatemala, right around the time of Rob's bathtub announcement, we hosted a huge baby-naming celebration at our home. The official reason for a Jewish baby-naming ceremony is to give a baby her Hebrew name. The unofficial reason was to show off our magnificent daughter to our community. I looked out at the familiar faces of the one hundred or so people who had come to help us welcome Dalia to the family. *We did it. All those years of wanting and pushing and trying and failing are behind us. We have two beautiful children, and before long we'll have a third. Nomi isn't here, and the presence of her absence will never go away, but here's Liat, smiling at me with Nomi's smile. And here's Dalia, whose middle name is Nomi.*

I saw Rachel looking at me proudly, holding her son Jake, and marveled at the way she and I, the two bookends to the threesome we once were, had become so much closer in the past few years. My dad, Rob, and Jonah, the unlikely three generations of males in my family, surrounded me. They came from different worlds and were now part of a lush and colorful family tree that for so many years I worried would remain barren. I took in the vases filled with dahlias I'd put on every shelf and windowsill and cleared my throat.

"Welcome everyone. Thank you so much for being here to help us celebrate Dalia," I said, as I hit the play button on my iPod. The rabbi, Jonah, Rob, and I stood at one end of the room, looking expectantly at the door where my mom and Dalia would enter.

My instructions to my mother had been clear: as soon as you hear the music start playing, carry Dalia into the room. I'd selected a gorgeous Hebrew song based on a biblical verse about journeying from one land to another, just as Dalia had from Guatemala City to Boston. The lyrics perfectly matched the promise of the day, and now as it rang out through the small portable speaker, I hoped it was having the same effect on the guests as it did for me each of the eighty-seven times I listened to it the night before.

I can't sing. I don't play an instrument. But listening to the right song at the right time makes me feel like Beyoncé playing a Stradivarius. I didn't hear it through my ears; I felt it in my body. This song, with its hopeful Hebrew words, part nostalgia, part optimism, felt like home. It was like a slice of chocolate pudding cake straight out of the oven—a dessert, a song, a day that was perfectly sweet and warmed my soul.

> *L'chi lach* [go forth], to a land that I will show you
> *Leich l'cha*, to a place you do not know
> *L'chi lach*, on your journey I will bless you
> And you shall be a blessing . . .

Everyone turned to look at the doorway, as though we were awaiting the bride's entrance.

But nothing happened.

"Where are they?" I whispered to Rob.

"I don't know. Should you go check?" he asked.

L'chi lach, and I shall make your name great
Leich l'cha, and all shall praise your name
L'chi lach, to the place that I will show you

The music continued to play.

"This is a little weird," I said out of the corner of my mouth. But then, just as I began to squeeze through the crowd to go find her, my mother waltzed into the room . . . literally. Far be it from Zelda to miss an opportunity to make a dramatic entrance. She twirled her way from the door to Rob and me. She took her time, cradling Dalia in one arm, the other raised above her head, moving in slow circles in time to the music. The guests parted, à la the Red Sea, to let them through.

I watched my mother carry my daughter and felt the love and hope they were radiating. And I knew, though most of the guests didn't, that she was celebrating not only Dalia, but also her own strength and happiness at being able to dance with her new granddaughter.

Three years earlier, right before we brought Jonah home from Guatemala, my mother was diagnosed with breast cancer. "It's going to be okay," she assured me when she called to tell me about the malignant lump. I was sobbing too hysterically to hear her. "Let me conference Rachel in," I whimpered, quickly tapping Rachel's number into the phone. I needed Rachel to be the mature one, to carry on the conversation and get all the details, so I could continue my bawling uninterrupted.

Ever since my sister Nomi died, I imagined, as vividly as I could stand to, the deaths of the people closest to me. I was so afraid of being caught off guard again that I wanted to be mentally prepared for losing someone else who was part of me. It was a stupid exercise at best, a twisted one at worst. Every time I considered what it might feel like to lose my mom, it felt like a hornet's nest exploded inside my stomach. I let myself feel it for a bare minute and then quickly changed the ruminations in my head to think about something less painful, like world hunger.

Now, a few years later, it seemed my mother had been right. It *was* okay. She'd endured multiple rounds of chemo and radiation. She'd lost her thick, frizzy hair and wore a sleek, silver wig, which we told her made her look like a Jewish Martha Stewart. She'd lost an alarming amount of weight when she couldn't eat and then gained more back when she became bloated from the meds. But now she had a clean bill of health. Now she was dancing with her new granddaughter, her own hair framing her beautiful face.

Feeling strong and infused with relief, she was able to throw herself more fully into grandmothering. She bought baskets filled with toys to keep at her apartment for the kids to play with when we visited, but all they wanted to do was sit next to her on the piano bench and tap the end of the keyboard while she played her Israeli music. When she came to our house, she occupied the kids with her gorilla imitation and silly voices while Rob cooked dinner and I folded laundry.

Relishing the role of Nani, she was thrilled when we told her we'd started the paperwork for baby number three.

Roberto was born nearly two years to the day after Dalia. It was somewhat perfect that his name was "Roberto," a cosmic wink to Rob that his namesake was waiting for us to come get him. But we needed to change his name, as it's against Jewish practice to name a child after a living relative. The theory goes that naming a child after someone who's still alive could appear as if you're expecting that person to die. God forbid the evil eye is watching and misinterprets.

But until we'd meet him and officially change his name, he was our little Roberto. We hung his picture on our refrigerator, so Jonah and Dalia would see him each day. He became somewhat of a family project, the missing puzzle piece that would complete us.

The desperation we felt when we were first waiting to become parents was gone. Jonah made us into parents. Dalia rounded us out. There was a family dynamic now, albeit a young one. Roberto would fit in rather than shape us.

"What should we name him?" we asked our kids. Jonah, now five, suggested "Señor Poopy Pants," but we didn't think that would go over well on his college applications. "What color should we paint his room?" "Pink!" Dalia said. "Should we get him a blanket with airplanes or one with cars?" "Pink bankie," she suggested. "Pink" was almost always Dalia's answer, no matter the question. My mother and I spent weeks moving around furniture to get a nursery ready for the new baby.

Then one Friday, I took the day off work, dropped the kids at the childcare center, and went to pick up my mom to take her for a follow-up with her oncologist. I'd taken her to the doctor dozens of times, and we had our routine down. I'd pick her up at her apartment and drive us to the hospital ten minutes away. We'd sit in the waiting room, Mom with her crossword puzzle and me with my *People* magazine. She'd ask me for a six-letter word that means "comestible;" I'd tell her who Brad Pitt might or might not be dating. During the actual appointment I'd take copious notes, recording everything the doctor said so I could share it with Rachel later. When it was all over, we'd go out to lunch. She'd have two glasses of chardonnay with her burger and fries. I'd get a turkey sandwich and a Diet Coke.

But this time was different. We knew it as soon as the doctor came into the room. There was no friendly banter, no beating around the bush.

He took a deep breath and began. "Here's what we're seeing. There's cancer in your bones. It's in your spine and your hip. We're going to need to do more scans and see if it's gone anywhere else." He went on for about ten minutes—tests and appointments and chemo and pain meds. He talked and I took notes and my mom listened stoically.

Zelda wasn't reserved in the slightest or reluctant to display her feelings in public. Quite the opposite, she relished big displays of emotion. Now I watched her carefully, her lips glued together, her eyes looking straight at the doctor. I couldn't get a read on what she was thinking. Maybe she was resigned or didn't understand the gravity of the news that was being delivered. She could have been in denial or figured she'd squash cancer this time like she did on the first go-round. Whatever the reason for her calm facade, I took my cues from her. If she was going to be so composed, I couldn't freak out in front of her.

I'd learned to save my sobbing for later.

When the doctor paused, my mom excused herself to go to the bathroom, opening a door for me I kind of preferred to keep closed.

"What does this mean?" I asked.

"Your mother is going to die from the breast cancer," he replied.

He was the one with the degrees on the wall, the one with dozens of people sitting in his waiting room, listening for their names to be called. And yet I thought this was a presumptuous decree for him to make. How did he know what my mother would die from? Maybe she'd be hit by a bus when we walked out of the hospital or be struck by lightning in a summer storm. *I'm not going to write this down*, I thought. *If I don't write it, maybe I can forget he said it.*

When my mom returned from the bathroom, we scheduled the follow-up appointments, went to the lab for blood draws, and headed out to lunch. As soon as we got in the car, I morphed into cheerleader mode. "Okay, so it's back," I started. "But we're going to beat this. You're the strongest person

I know, and you will tell this fucking cancer who's boss." I wasn't used to my mother's silence, and I compensated for it by continuing to talk, picking up my pace as I went. "We did it before and we'll do it again. It's going to be fine. It sucks, but we'll get through it."

Filling the space with my words, I made promises I had no right to make.

Years later I'd learn how to sit quietly in sadness. But at that time admitting despair was akin to admitting defeat. I was still rambling as we entered the restaurant, still blathering on when the waitress came to take our order. "I'll have a chardonnay," my mother said. "Me, too," I said, understanding that a Diet Coke wasn't going to cut it.

"Darling, let's talk about the baby," my mother said. I told her we'd narrowed down the names to Theo, Max, or Noah, though we were concerned that together Noah and Jonah would sound too aquatic. I pulled out his picture, and together we marveled at his delicious thighs, his contagious smile. We ordered refills on our chardonnays and started planning the party we'd have when we brought our baby home.

7

Fly Away

Five months later, my mother was admitted to the hospital for the last time.

The cancer was in her brain, in her colon, and throughout her bones. She'd shrunk all over, like she was clanking around inside the body that just a few months ago had seemed too small to contain her.

"She's not eating at all," the doctor told me. "That's a sign that she's nearing the end."

"Then I'll get her to eat," I said, because mind over matter. I sat by her bedside and tried to spoon-feed her applesauce. It was such an obvious role reversal it almost felt cliché. I bit my tongue so I wouldn't ask her to open wide for the choo-choo train, like I did when I fed Jonah and Dalia.

And then she looked at me with eyes that had become slightly too big for their sockets and said, "Don't. Force. Me. To. Eat." Her mouth was so dry it was a bit hard to understand her, but she said it so slowly and so emphatically that I heard what she said and, as always with my mother, what she didn't. She was done. "You have to eat, Mom. You have to eat. Please eat." But she'd fallen asleep. Rachel came into the room just then to take over. I handed her the spoon as I quickly gathered my purse and my jacket. "Make her eat."

The phone rang early the next day. "Jessie, it's Jane. Good news! We just found out they're ready for you to come sign the paperwork for Roberto. I know it's really short notice, but is there any way you and Rob can be in Guatemala next week?"

Guatemala? Next week? What about my mom? What about feeding her applesauce? What about willing her to get better?

"Jane, my mother is really, really sick. I'm not sure I can leave her right now. Is there any way Rob could go alone and take care of the paperwork?" I asked, not having the slightest idea how Rob would feel about this proposition.

"I'm so sorry to hear about your mother, truly I am. But Jessie, Guatemala is really close to a complete shutdown for adoptions. You both need to go now if you're going to adopt Roberto."

I called my mother's doctor to explain our dilemma. I was looking for reassurance, but he wasn't playing.

"I can't tell you what to do, but I can't promise that your mother will make it until you get back."

Our family, now almost complete, was also falling apart.

It was a milder version of Sophie's choice, an impossible decision. Roberto was our child, just as much as Jonah and Dalia. We'd committed our hearts to him. But I knew the doctors thought my mother was going to die soon. I couldn't abandon her.

I went upstairs to Jonah's room and found Rob cuddled in bed reading with both kids.

It was *The Runaway Bunny*, one of the staples in our repertoire. I listened from the doorway, marveling at the way the kids were tucked perfectly into Rob's arms, one on each side.

In the story, the bunny wants to set out on her own, teasing her mother with all the ways she could leave.

I'd never even particularly liked this book, but now it seemed like it was written solely to twist my knotted stomach even tighter.

Was I the bunny, sailing away from my mother?

The mother counters each threat with a promise that she'll always be with the bunny, even if she needs to become the wind or a tightrope walker to get to her.

Oh shit, maybe I'm the mother who's supposed to walk across the air to Roberto.

"What's wrong, Mommy?" Jonah asked.

"Nothing, sweetie. I'm fine," I said, wiping the tears from my cheeks.

"Why you so sad, Mama?" Dalia's question made the tears come more quickly.

I gave the kids my "I'm-trying-to-hide-my-sadness-and-not-upset-you-with-what's-really-going-on-but-we-all-know-you-can-see-right-through-that" smile. My tears were a giveaway.

"I'll be back in a minute," Rob said to the kids.

We sat on the floor in the hallway, our backs against the wall.

"Sweetyheart," he began. "We'll do whatever you want. If you aren't comfortable leaving your mom, we'll find a way to convince the agency to let us wait."

"I don't think we can. It really seems like Jane was saying it's now or never."

"It's your call," he said. "I'm not going to tell you to leave your mother right now. I want us to go, and we can do it as quickly as possible, but if you're not okay with that, then we should stay."

If he pressured me to go, I knew I wouldn't be able to forgive him if my mother died while we were gone, and he knew that too. But I also hated that he was leaving it up to me. What if we stayed and lost Roberto?

I called Rachel, who had a childhood's worth of experience telling me what to do.

"Jess, you need to go meet your baby," she said without hesitating. "Mom will be okay. I'll be with her, and we'll call you every hour if you want us to. You can come right back if we need you."

We went to Guatemala for thirty-six hours to meet Roberto and sign the papers that would allow us to adopt him four months later.

I hated flying back then. I kept a catalogue of past plane crashes in my head—the one where the pilot forgot to deice the wings, the one where a bird flew into the engine, the one where the plane skidded into the harbor after landing. But this time I forgot to be afraid of crashing. I was too busy being afraid that my mother would die while we were in the air.

Trying to focus on what we were heading toward instead of what we were leaving behind, I pulled out the stack of pictures I'd brought with me. The top three were of Roberto, his smile taking up half of each photo, his thighs taking up the other. The rest of the pictures were ones I'd carefully chosen of Dalia to share with her birth mother, Ana. The Guatemalan lawyer who handled our adoptions had told Ana we were coming to town, and she'd asked if she could visit with us.

I wasn't threatened by the idea of Ana—or the reality of Ana—anymore. I didn't yet believe as I do now that Ana and I were cosmically connected. She brought Dalia into the world, and I was ushering her through it. On that trip it felt more like Ana was a distant relative to whom we were paying our respects when we came to town.

We were on a condensed timetable, so we went straight from the airport to the hotel lobby for the meeting. We stood up when we saw our translator Oscar walk in. Ana and her mother were a few paces behind. Had they not been together, we might not have recognized Ana. Slim when we first met, she was now gaunt, walking ever so slowly and leaning on her mother for support.

We spent the next hour huddled around a table in the corner of the lobby. We shared the pictures and told them how Dalia looked up to Jonah and giggled at *Boohbah* on TV and slept with a stuffed animal she called Squiddie. We wanted them to know that Dalia was happy and that she made everyone around her happy too.

As they were leaving, I pulled Oscar aside.

"Ana looks so different. Is she okay?"

"I'm not sure," he said quietly. "They don't know what's wrong, but they think it's something with her stomach."

We never could have imagined then that her illness would one day define everything about our lives.

– ≫ ≪ –

I talked to Rachel eight times while we were in Guatemala. She held the phone to my mother's ear, and I gave her the play-by-play of everything that was happening.

I told her about Ana, and then I told her about Theo.

"He's twenty-two pounds of pure joy," I told her. "He's just so huge and happy. He's twice as big as any of the other babies we've seen around the hotel. I actually feel kind of bad for the other parents because their babies look so sad and squirmy in comparison. You're going to love him, Mom."

One week after we got back from Guatemala, my mother died. The hornet nest exploded in my stomach, and the hornets had sharp quills that traveled through me, jabbing every inch of my intestines. Imagining the worst thing doesn't make you any more prepared when it happens.

I stood between Rachel and Rob at the funeral, trying to listen to the rabbi's words, but the rushing in my ears drowned out everything. I stood at the podium, holding hands with Rachel as we gave a eulogy of our own, but I felt more like I was playing the part of the grieving daughter than actually being the grieving daughter. Because how could any of this be real? How could my mother, more full of life than anyone I knew, be gone? I stood to recite the words of the Twenty-

Third Psalm, "Yea though I walk through the valley of the shadow of death, I will fear no evil: for Thou art with me; Thy rod and Thy staff they comfort me." But I found no comfort in either the rod or the staff. And then I stood and watched as Rob and my brother-in-law David walked on either side of my mother's casket, escorting her to the waiting hearse. The words of the song I insisted the funeral director play, even though he said it was against their custom to play recorded music at a funeral, rang out.

> *L'chi lach*, to a land that I will show you
> *Leich l'cha*, to a place you do not know
> *L'chi lach*, on your journey I will bless you
> And you shall be a blessing… *l'chi lach*

I closed my eyes and saw my mother dancing into the room with Dalia at the baby naming. The words that felt so perfect then felt even more so now. And I knew that if there was such a thing as heaven or any kind of life after life, my mother and Nomi were dancing together now.

PART TWO

We All Fall Down

8

Quieting the Disquiet

That first summer as a family of five, we went to visit Rob's parents at their cottage in Canada. I'd been to the cottage a dozen times before, but this was the first time I was looking forward to it. The fact that there was so little to do there finally appealed to me. Plus, I was now bringing the grand prize. I was thirty-nine years old. I'd published a book in my twenties, wrote a weekly column for a major newspaper, and was a vice president of the global company where I'd worked for a decade. But all that time I was busy succeeding in one aspect of my life, I'd been failing at another.

Each time we visited Rob's parents during all those years of failed baby making, I felt like we were arriving empty-handed. Now, I'd be showing up at my in-laws' home with three kids in tow, an abundance of riches. Jonah, Dalia, and Theo would play with the toys that previously mocked us from their place on the shelves. I'd hear my mother-in-law's stories about raising three children with appreciation and camaraderie. I'd nod knowingly, rather than longingly. Plus, I was desperate for a nap, and I knew Rob and my mother-in-law, Barb, would happily watch the kids and let me sleep.

I am woman; hear me roar, I thought, walking across the tarmac balancing baby Theo in one arm and Dalia, now three, in the other.

In the rustic living room of the cottage, Barb, Dalia, and her crusty baby blanket, Stinky Lovie, cuddled together while Barb read *How Much Is That Doggie in the Window?* for the sixth time in a row. "Ga!" Dalia said, as soon as Barb finished the story. "Again?" Barb repeated, understanding that "ga" was how Dalia pronounced "again."

I sat at the kitchen table nearby, drinking a glass of wine and looking out the window at Jonah, Rob, and my father-in-law by the lake. Theo perched beside them, filling and emptying buckets of sand. There was a stone-skipping contest happening, and Jonah was winning. It was so peaceful, so *On Golden Pond*-esque. *I could spend the whole summer here*, I thought, as I topped off my glass of wine.

"Okay, Dalia, time for Grandma to make dinner," Barb said, extricating herself from Dalia and Stinky Lovie. Dalia slid off the couch and began to make her way over to me, putting one of her hands on the wall to steady herself as she walked the twelve steps to my lap. "Dal, let's go see the boys," I said, scooping her up and heading out the door straight for the beach.

The next morning, the seven of us went blueberry picking. In my entire life before I met Rob, I'd never done anything that felt as wholesome. The closest I had come to blueberry picking was in the produce section of the grocery store. It wasn't just that we were going to an actual field to pick actual blueberries, it was that later that afternoon the kids would help Barb make blueberry crumble and blueberry pie from scratch. I'd never baked a pie with my grandmother, or with my mother for that matter, and it seemed like the kind of thing one does in the Rockwellian childhood I suddenly seemed to be providing for my children.

After we unpacked ourselves from the van at the edge of the field, Rob handed out the pails and then took off with his father and Jonah. Barb held Theo's hand as he waddled slightly in front of her. I'm not sure if he was more excited about the fact that he recently mastered walking and there was an endless runway in front of him or that as far as he could see there were plump blueberries for the taking. Dalia took just a couple of steps before plopping down on her knees and beginning to fill her bucket.

I watched as she put three berries in her mouth for each one that went in the pail. *That takes strength, right?* I thought. *Some of those berries need a good tug to break loose. It looks like she's using small motor skills. The berries are ending up exactly where she wants them to go. And she's so focused. Maybe everybody's right. Maybe it's just going to take her a little longer to catch up.*

At first, Dalia hit all the standard milestones—rolling over, pushing up, toddling. We were told at every well-visit (kids' checkups are referred to as "well-visits," which looking back today seems improbably optimistic) that she was on track and developing normally.

But there was a gnawing feeling, an insistent whisper in my head that something wasn't right. Dalia's toddling didn't evolve into a more assured gait, as I'd seen happen with my kids' friends. Instead, she remained wobbly—as though she were always walking in a bit of a drunken stupor. And when she began to speak, her words sounded garbled.

I'd been working on being a relaxed parent, trying to find the right balance between not hovering so closely the kids couldn't fall and being there to pick them up when the fall was a bad one.

But any outward expression of relaxation didn't quiet the disquiet in my head. *Was this normal?* It was totally different from what we experienced with Jonah, who was on the go from the first day we met him. And even though he didn't hear English as a baby, he mastered the basics quickly and spoke in easily decipherable sentences early on. I knew it wasn't a good idea to compare one child to another, but there was empirical data living in our house that was impossible for me to ignore.

Rob, on the other hand, didn't need to work at all on being relaxed. Being outwardly calm was his natural state, with any nascent fears or anxieties kept tucked firmly inside. Midwest stock versus East Coast perhaps, Protestant compared to Jew. He'd converted and was now Jewish, too, but his restrained composition hadn't been washed away by the mikvah. The ritual immersion in a pool of natural water marked his conversion but didn't change his constitution.

A year earlier my friend Olivia told me about Early Intervention, a state program that provides services for children under three with developmental delays. "It's awesome," she told me, as we watched our kids doing varied facsimiles of somersaults in their Little Tumblers class. "Sam's made progress already, and it's only been two months."

I figured I had nothing to lose by scheduling a screening. Olivia told me a couple of therapists would come to the house and play games with Dalia for a few hours. If they identified any delays, we'd qualify for free services—physical or speech therapy of some sort.

A few weeks later I lurked nearby while the specialists played blocks and colored with Dalia, hoping that what looked like ordinary activities to me were uncovering profound insights for them.

"Dalia is a delightful child," one of the therapists reported back a few hours later. *Here it comes*, I thought. *Start with the delightful personality to cushion the blow.* "Her large and small motor functions are both within the low-normal range. Kids develop at different speeds, and we really don't have any information about what her diet was like during the first months of her life or how much stimulation she got. Both of those variables could account for her being on the lower end of average. Give it a few months and she'll almost definitely catch up."

A few weeks later, I got a call from the director at Dalia's childcare center. "Dalia fell while carrying her tray to the sink. She's okay, but she has a pretty big egg on her forehead." I got a similar call a few weeks later and then another a month after that.

I called Early Intervention a second time and asked them to come back. This time they played new, more advanced games. "Dalia doesn't meet the criteria for services," they reported. "She's still within the normal range."

How many falls will it take for her to qualify? I wondered, glancing at the lingering bruise on Dalia's forehead. I'd initially called Early Intervention to be reassured Dalia was okay, but that very reassurance felt like a major miscalculation.

Now, I noticed how intently Dalia focused on the blueberries. Every few minutes she swatted one of her long, thick black pigtails off her face, leaving a smear of blueberry juice across her cheek. Her skin had darkened in the thirty minutes we'd been sitting in the field. She now looked more maple than pecan. She squeezed her eyes shut every minute or so, likely as a respite from the hot sun, but the movement only accentuated the obscene length of her eyelashes and the fact that she'd likely never feel compelled to wear mascara.

She looked up and saw me watching her. "Mama, where my Fio?" she asked. From the moment we brought Theo home, Dalia believed we added him to the family specifically for her benefit. He wasn't so much a toy for her to play with as a baby for her to mother. She held his bottle at mealtime, rubbed his back in his crib, and hugged him in her lap on the couch.

"Let's go find him," I said, taking her hand and the pail, letting the beauty of the day suffocate the ruminations in my head.

9

If I Knew Then

Weekday mornings were the most hectic time of the week. I did whatever it took to get the kids to cooperate. I bribed. I counted. I yelled. I begged. Getting the three of them dressed and fed, their teeth and hair passably brushed, so that I could drop Jonah at the bus stop and the other two at the childcare center in time to get to work for my morning meeting was always an iffy proposition. One cranky toddler, one nap mat that didn't make it from the washing machine to the dryer could be the difference between arriving at work in time to get a decent parking space and a cup of coffee before gracefully walking into my boss's office or dashing in, coat still on, apologizing as I wiped the muffin crumbs from my face and dug my computer out of my briefcase.

One morning, when Dalia was four, we were already running ten minutes late when I realized her left shoe had disappeared.

"Sweetie," I said in my let's-try-patience-first voice. "Run upstairs and get your shoe please." She turned and made her way to the stairs—no whining, no dawdling. But then she got on all fours and began to make the ascent, crablike, alternating hands and knees, right and then left, ever so slowly.

"Can you move a little faster, please," I shouted as I zipped up Theo's jacket.

"No, Mom, she can't," said Jonah.

I looked at him, standing by the door, absentmindedly twirling his Rubik's Cube. He wasn't being a smart ass. He suspected, as I did, that Dalia was moving as fast as she could.

I turned and looked at Dalia, who'd finished her climb and found her shoe. I watched as she began to slide down the stairs on her bottom. And I made a mental note to add "call the pediatrician" to my to-do list.

They say mother's intuition is a real thing, that mothers have a sixth sense that alerts them to the state of their children's well-being. We've all heard stories of parents who respond to a gut feeling, turning just in time to pull a hand from a flame or calling to check in with the babysitter right as a major temper tantrum is erupting.

Was it mother's intuition that wouldn't let me believe Dalia was fine even though all the experts said she was? If mother's intuition is a biological response, as some data uggest, could it be a thing for adoptive mothers?

Later that day, I was in my office reviewing cover photos for a new parent brochure. The first picture was of three babies seated next to each other on the floor, cracking up. They looked like little old men, with their bald heads, protruding bellies, and crinkled eyes. It was impossible not to smile when looking at them, to wonder what was making them laugh so deliciously. The second was of two toddlers, playing together in a sandbox. One of the kids was shoveling sand into a pail the other was holding. In the background was a teacher, observing the kids but not interrupting them. It was a great depiction of child-led play and teamwork. I came to the third option: a preschool-age girl in a bright red dress running through a puddle while hugging a big yellow rubber ball. Her black pigtails fluttered behind her as she flew across the page. If I squinted, the blurry girl was Dalia boldly dashing through the storm. I looked at the picture for ten minutes, imagining my daughter, graceful and fearless. *Will she ever feel that confident? Will I?*

I shut the door and called the pediatrician.

"Things haven't gotten better. Dalia's constantly off-balance. She's falling more and more. Something isn't right."

"What are you afraid of?" he asked.

"I'm afraid there's something wrong in her brain," I answered, realizing as I heard myself that I was afraid there was something wrong in her brain.

"Well, we don't have any reason to believe that's the case," he said, "but we've talked about this long enough, and I agree we should do some tests. Let's get a workup with an audiologist. Maybe her balance issues are inner-ear related."

The call came soon after the hearing test, while I was in the middle of preparing five bagged lunches for the next day.

"Dalia has a mild to moderate high-frequency sensorineural permanent hearing loss, which means she has trouble hearing high-pitched sounds," the doctor said.

"Okay. What can we do about that? How do we fix it?" I asked, pushing the question around the tennis ball that had settled in my throat. I reached for a pen to write down what he was saying. "Hearing loss," I scribbled quickly, showing the piece of paper to Rob.

"It can't be cured, but we can address it with hearing aids, and we should be able to restore all the sounds she's missing. I think we'll see a big improvement in her speech and maybe even her balance once she can hear better."

What I heard the doctor say was this: Dalia is going to need hearing aids. My stomach clenched as I imagined kids on the playground making fun of her.

Even though hearing loss was worlds better than being told there was something wrong in Dalia's brain, I still felt nauseous. Now there was an actual diagnosis, and it scared me. My fear overpowered any sense of relief I might have felt.

My friends were sympathetic. "Jess, I'm so, so sorry. But at least there's something that can be done about it," Lara said. "My daughter has a friend with hearing aids," my friend Sue told me. "Do you want me to have her come meet you and Dalia?" "Poor Dalia," Rachel said. "Is there anything I can do to cheer her up?" My father moved immediately into research mode. "I've been reading about cochlear implants. Let's find out if that's an option for us. Let's see if there's a study we can get her into. Let's find the most esteemed hearing doctor in the world."

Nobody told me what I would now tell my younger self: "Bedazzle the heck out of the hearing aids, and start learning American Sign Language ASAP. Get a grip. In the grand scheme of things, it could be a whole lot worse."

And if anyone *had* told me those things, I wouldn't have listened. Perspective is a gift most of us are only given in hindsight; it can't be force-fed. And just because things could have been—and would in fact turn out to be—much worse, the hearing loss diagnosis was no small thing.

Yet now I know that a diagnosis that can be corrected with a nonintrusive device like hearing aids isn't a life changer. I know that hearing aids are essentially just another accessory, no different from glasses. And most of all, now I know that I would give my limbs to have the only thing wrong with Dalia be mild to moderate hearing loss.

10

The Decree

Dalia's big eyes and dainty mouth both opened wide when the audiologist put in the hearing aids for the first time. "Can you hear this?" the audiologist asked, pressing play on her tape recorder. Dalia nodded. Rob and I watched in amazement. "Tank you, Mama and Daddy," Dalia said with a huge smile as we left the office. In the car, we made up a new game where I said words from the driver's seat for Dalia to repeat. I softened my voice as we played, like the auditory version of the shrinking lines on an eye chart.

"Flower," I shouted.

"Flower," she shouted back.

"Party," I said.

"Party," she repeated.

"Ice cream," I whispered.

"My hungry! My want ice cream!"

I'd wasted so much energy worrying. Dalia was excited about her "ear helpers," which was a term we all liked better than hearing aids. We found a purple sparkly pair that was kind of cool, and other than the fact that she flushed one of them down the toilet just six weeks after she started wearing them, the pros of the hearing aids far outweighed the cons I imagined.

But her speech and balance issues didn't improve. If anything, they seemed more exaggerated. Every morning, when we piled out of the car at the childcare center, Theo and I stood on either side of Dalia, each holding one of her hands. "What's gonna work? Teamwork!" we sang, putting our singular spin on the theme song of *Wonder Pets*, a family favorite at the time. But really it was a way for the two of us to steady Dalia as we walked across the parking lot, clutching her hands to prevent a wipeout on the asphalt.

There was still the burning question of what caused the hearing loss. Was it structural? Genetic? Related to an infection she had as an infant? Did it matter?

"Let's do a genetic workup," the doctor suggested. "It's a simple blood draw, and it might let us rule out some possible causes for the hearing loss." Maybe we'd get some answers, a reason for the delays, the balance issues, and the hearing loss. And if there was an explanation, presumably there'd be a treatment.

We went to the hospital for the blood tests and then to Ben & Jerry's for banana splits, because clearly the former is deserving of the latter.

"How nervous should we be?" I asked Rob that night. I'd asked that very question of Rob many times before and have asked it hundreds of times since, his response giving me a barometer of how much anxiety I might have needlessly created versus how much is actually called for. It's a trick that usually calms me right down, given that Rob is always less nervous than I am.

"I don't think we need to be too scared," he assured me. "It's just a way for us to get more information. And you know she's rocking those hearing aids."

— ›› ‹‹ —

When a doctor calls and asks you to come to his office to discuss test results in person, it's usually not a good thing, and in fact it's probably a really bad thing. I knew enough to have my father come with us when the doctor said we needed to come in and Dalia didn't need to be at the appointment. We needed someone adultier than we were.

The three of us, the doctor, and a genetic counselor squeezed into a tiny exam room. There weren't enough chairs for all of us, yet we didn't even lean on the empty exam table, keeping it and the clean white paper that covered it pristine out of an unspoken respect for the little girl we were discussing.

The doctor, whom we'd never met before, jumped right in. "I'm afraid the blood tests surfaced a diagnosis for your daughter," he started. "Dalia tested positive for a genetic mutation that's associated with MERRF syndrome, myoclonic epilepsy with ragged red fibers, a rare form of mitochondrial disease."

We'd never heard of MERRF syndrome. I *had* heard of mitochondria, had a vague recollection of the word from tenth-grade biology class, though I had no idea what they were or why we needed them.

"What do the mitochondria do?" my father asked, swallowing audibly and putting his arm around me.

"Mitochondria are the powerhouse of the body's cells, responsible for converting protein into energy," the doctor said. "Every organ relies on mitochondria to function properly, so if your mitochondria aren't working like they're supposed to, neither can your body."

He pulled out human body models. He showed us diagrams. He talked and talked, and I heard less and less of what he was saying.

I didn't understand what it all meant. I wanted to ask: *What in the world are you talking about? Have you seen our perfect daughter?*

I began to tune out the doctor, focusing not on his words, but instead on mental images of Dalia playing with her brothers, dancing to Katy Perry, snuggling in bed as I read her a story. I couldn't comprehend what he was telling us, couldn't reconcile the black-and-white diagrams he showed with the vibrant filmstrip of Dalia running through my head.

"Do we know how she got this?" my father asked. Rob and I were holding hands, and I was trying to take notes with my free hand, but it was shaking and the words I wrote were nearly illegible.

"MERRF is almost always maternally inherited." He took a long breath. "There's one other piece of information I need you to understand."

He looked at me, glanced at Rob, then back to me. "This disease is degenerative, and there's no cure."

Most of the appointment was a blur, but that word stuck out and echoed in my head: "degenerative."

We were silent, lost in our own confusion.

Then my dad spoke up. "How quickly will things get worse?"

"That's the thing about a rare disease," the doctor said. "There's just not enough information for us to rely on. There isn't a large enough data sample to help us predict the course and speed of progression. But in the areas where she's already showing symptoms, her symptoms will get worse. For example, the fact that she's having balance issues now means she'll most likely need a wheelchair."

I looked at the tendons bulging on Rob's neck before squeezing my eyes shut. I tried to block out the doctor and the room and the words coming out of his mouth.

"How soon? Are you sure?" Rob pressed.

"I'm guessing it will happen by the time she's in third grade," the doctor said quietly.

Her speech and motor issues meant it was likely she'd have brain degeneration, too, he explained. We didn't press him on that one. My stomach clenched and my palms began sweating, so maybe my body was hearing what he was saying, but my brain couldn't accept it. It was simply inconceivable.

Afterward, we were quiet in the crowded elevator. I leaned against the back wall as we descended, needing the support to keep from disintegrating. Rob's shoulders slumped. His eyes fixed on the glowing orange numbers changing in front of us. On the wall next to the elevator door was a sign that read, "In case of emergency, push alarm." I wanted so badly to push that button. I wanted bells to go off and sirens to ring and people in uniform to rush in and do something to make this disaster go away.

Back in the lobby, Rob gave me a hug and said, "We're going to figure this out. It's going to be okay." I didn't know which one of us he was trying to convince, and I didn't care, because his words were a balm. He left to pick up the kids.

I turned to my dad and said, "I'm just glad we didn't know."

I was glad Dalia hadn't been diagnosed with MERRF syndrome at birth. If she had, if we had been told about a baby girl available for adoption with a rare degenerative disease, I wouldn't have been prepared or interested in taking on that kind of challenge. I would have simply passed, and we never would have met our daughter. I was the one who didn't want to check any of the boxes on the list of "acceptable medical conditions" years before.

I feel like a bit of an imposter when I meet people now who tell us they think we're "amazing" or "inspiring"—assuming, I guess, that we found out about a little girl with severe needs and adopted her. We aren't the ones you read about in *People* magazine who adopt twelve kids with special needs. We're not even the ones who spend every weekend preparing and delivering warm meals to homeless people. Those people are amazing. We're the ones who are just like so many others—the ones who got dealt a horrible blow and who try every day to do our best to rise to the occasion.

I was glad we hadn't known, because by the time Dalia was diagnosed, she was ours and we were hers. She couldn't have been any more my daughter if she had had my healthy genes coursing through her body.

At home, I went straight to my computer and searched for MERRF syndrome. The National Organization of Rare Diseases defined it this way:

> MERRF (*m*yoclonus *e*pilepsy with *r*agged-*r*ed *f*ibers) syndrome is an extremely rare disorder that begins in childhood and affects the nervous system and skeletal muscle as well as other body systems. Individuals with MERRF syndrome may have muscle weakness (myopathy), an impaired ability to coordinate movements (ataxia), seizures, and a slow deterioration of intellectual function (dementia). Short stature, degeneration of the optic nerve (optic atrophy), hearing loss, cardiomyopathy and abnormal sensation from nerve damage (peripheral neuropathy) are also common symptoms.

Reading all this together was simply too much to integrate. The description felt so different from Dalia, so removed from our reality. It was like I was reading the small print at the bottom of an ad for Tylenol, the possible side effects that nobody thinks are actually going to happen.

I made two phone calls. The first was to my brother-in-law David. Given that he was a doctor and the best diagnostician I knew, he might have some useful insights. Instead, he expressed his sympathy and lovingly suggested I speak with a therapist. It wasn't the reassurance I'd hoped for.

The second was to the adoption agency. We now suspected what made Dalia's birth mother sick. Given that MERRF was so rare, we were nearly certain she hadn't been diagnosed in Guatemala. If we could give her this information, maybe she'd be able to treat her symptoms. But the agency and their network in Guatemala couldn't find her.

We never found out what happened to Dalia's birth mother, but I think of her from time to time. I wonder how ill she became from MERRF and whether she ever found out what was wrong with her. I think of all we owed her for entrusting us with Dalia, and once in a while I allow myself to wonder how things would have unfolded had Dalia stayed in Guatemala.

But that evening, after calling the adoption agency, I wasn't thinking about Dalia's birth mother. I was thinking about Dalia and how surreal the diagnosis felt. When we were struggling with infertility, Rachel compared it to walking through your life with an umbrella over your head. You might go to work or to a party or to the movies, you might forget for a little while, but there's always a bit of a dark shadow with you. Now, with this new diagnosis, the doctor had handed us another umbrella. The shadow was more ominous, but it was also a lot murkier. How could feisty, sweet, funny Dalia have a rare degenerative disease? It made no sense.

That night, we had Dalia's favorite foods for dinner: dinosaur-shaped chicken nuggets, french fries, and chocolate cake. We let Dalia dig into the cake with her hands, because why not? After dinner, we decided to play hide-and-seek. Dalia and I were on the same team, as always. Jonah was "It," and as we heard him start counting down from ten, Dalia said, "Mama, we go to your bathroom." "Great idea," I said, walking behind her, my hands under her arms to keep her steady. When we got to the bathroom, I lifted Dalia into our tub and crouched down, hugging her in front of me. Somehow while crouching, my back nudged the faucet.

Water began pouring out of the rain showerhead we had installed earlier that year, soaking both of us. Fleetingly I thought, *How fucking fitting.* I quickly moved to lift Dalia out of the tub, but I could see that she was laughing so hard she was crying. It was impossible to tell her tears from the water. I settled back down, hugged Dalia tighter, and laughed along with her, the water washing over both of us. "I guess you don't need a bath tonight, sweetie," I said.

We were given life-changing news, but our lives hadn't changed. In the morning I'd head to Arizona for a business trip, and I'd spend the entire flight reading about mitochondria and rare diseases. I'd step out of my meetings to leave messages for the doctors the geneticist told us about. I'd come home a day early because it didn't feel good to be away and because

I felt like I had a legitimate excuse to cut the trip short. But that night there were games to play, baths to ignore, and extra snuggles to steal, all of which felt much more real and much more urgent than this lurking disease that was just starting to emerge from the shadows.

11

Sinking and Soaring

By kindergarten, Dalia needed a walker. By the end of first grade, she used a wheelchair when she had to walk more than a few steps. "Mama, why my legs no work like they're supposed to?" Dalia asked.

"Oh, sweetie, different bodies work different ways," I fumbled. "Jonah's eyes need help, so he wears glasses. Your legs need help. They get tired and that makes it hard to walk sometimes." It was insufficient and not at all what I wanted to say, which was, "Because life is unfair, and you got dealt a shitty hand, and I wish I could give you my legs."

The medications she took each day increased as we tried to manage the symptoms of her weakening muscles. We gave her compounded high doses of vitamins and supplements to compensate for the deterioration, mixing them with applesauce and pudding to mask the horrible smell. "Gusting," Dalia said, letting us know we hadn't succeeded. Rob sampled the vitamins, to see firsthand how bad it really was. "It is gusting," he agreed. We doubled the amount of applesauce and pudding.

Rob and I had a "business meeting" every Sunday night, where we went over the coming week's schedule and figured out who could miss work for what, because now tossed in with Jonah's tae kwon do and baseball and Theo's clarinet lesson and fencing class, we had Dalia's speech therapy and physical therapy and regular appointments with the orthopedist, the ophthalmologist, the audiologist, and the neurologist. It felt like a heartbreaking game of chicken, or maybe chess, as we puzzled over who could miss work when. "If I do the Tuesday appointment, can you take Friday morning?"

I did my best to understand what I'd failed to learn in high school—how cells work and energy functions. There wasn't much to read on MERRF syndrome*—and what I did read I wished I hadn't. Every article said the symptoms could vary widely. There was a long list of possible manifestations, so I chose to believe that while she had the muscle twitches, weakness, and hearing loss, she'd be spared the blindness and dementia. If I thought for even a minute about Dalia losing her sight or suffering from dementia, the blood in my arms burned and my fingers tingled. I started to sweat and feel queasy, so I tried to push those possibilities out of my mind. It was like that clunking noise you hear when you turn a corner in the car. Ignore it long enough, maybe it will go away.

Most of the time, my strategy worked. I rarely fell apart or secretly cried on the bathroom floor. I didn't skip work to stay in bed and perseverate on "what ifs." I just kept moving forward. Keeping busy with all the logistics and research was a perfect way to avoid dealing with the fear and sadness. Over time the to-do list became a suit of armor, a complete body

*Author's note: Today, if you google MERRF syndrome, one of the first images that comes up is a photo of Dalia. She has become part of the definition of the disease.

harness to protect me from crumbling under the weight of despair.

But the emotions were always pressing against the armor, and sometimes they broke free.

– »» «« –

Rob and I circled around each other, feeling out our new roles. Sometimes he did the hands-on work while I cheered him on. Other times I took the lead, using the organizational skills I'd mastered in the corporate world to keep our world spinning. Romance wasn't just put on the back burner; it was packed up in a box and stored in the basement.

We decided to invest in a regular Saturday night date night. Every week, as soon as we got into the car, one of us would say, "We've never needed a date more." And every week we meant it. The kids loved this arrangement, too, because they got to spend the evening with our babysitter, Kim, who was way more fun than we were.

One Saturday night, we were at our favorite restaurant. Rob was perusing the beer selection and I was deciding between the cabernet and merlot, when out of nowhere, I began sobbing– shoulders heaving, nose running, the whole thing.

"Sweetyheart, what's going on? Do you feel sick?" Rob asked. "Do you want to leave?"

I was just as surprised as Rob by my tears.

"I can't believe I'm never going to have a 'girls' day' with a teenage Dalia. I just want to be able to do all the things I did with my mother—go out to lunch and to the movies and for long walks around the reservoir. I want to drop her off at college and help her pick a wedding dress."

Dalia was seven at the time.

"You'll have girls' days," Rob said. "They'll just look a little bit different. Everything's just going to look a little bit different."

"But I don't want them to look different," I hiccuped.

I wanted Rob to reassure me. I wanted him to tell me that of course Dalia and I would do all those things. I wanted him to tell me, as he had hundreds of times before, that my fears were unfounded. Instead, he held my hand across the table and ordered our drinks.

Weeks later, Rob would admit that the thing he mourned in advance was someday walking Dalia down the aisle at her wedding. He wanted to join with his brothers in lifting Dalia and the person she'd marry in wobbly chairs overhead while the wedding guests danced around them. "Like they lifted us at our wedding," he said. "I want to see her that happy."

But that night he let the grieving be mine. It would be too painful for us to be there together.

By Monday, I was back in research mode, searching for experimental treatments, for clinical trials, for reasons to be hopeful.

Part of it was wanting to feel like we were being proactive. Ever since I became a mother in a hotel room in Guatemala City, my first priority was to keep my children safe and healthy.

And if I couldn't do that, I was failing. This was beyond nursing a fever or installing a car seat or making sure the bike helmet fit properly. Those things had quickly become JV.

I had a secret fantasy that I'd be the one to come up with a cure for MERRF. I knew how to get things done, how to make things happen. So what if I'd only recently learned what mitochondria do? I imagined there'd one day be a movie made in the vein of *Lorenzo's Oil*. *Dalia's Tincture*, or something like that. I'd find the brilliant young scientist, the weed with medicinal properties, the precise combination of diet and exercise that cured damaged mitochondria.

I knew we were in a race against time. Dalia was learning and growing. We were practicing sight words with her, and she could read the basic board books that spilled out of her bookshelf. She could write decipherable words. I'd find notes in my workbag that said, "I love you Mama. Love Dalia." The notes always had a colorful rainbow taking up most of the page. And she was so eager to swallow up every new bit of learning. "My do it," she'd say, when we moved to help her put on her shoes or tried to steady her trembling hand when she was brushing her teeth.

But for every new development, there were also the things that were becoming harder. We were trying to cram as much knowledge and growth into Dalia as possible to outweigh all that was slipping away. Because even though the doctors hadn't been able to give us a precise timeline, we knew that Dalia was learning and losing simultaneously.

I read everything I could find online about mitochondrial studies or research and wrote letters to the doctors and scientists whose names appeared at the bottom of the page. I became addicted to googling, trying every key word I could think of, reluctant to skip even a day in case I missed the announcement of a new treatment or an experimental trial.

And in the meantime, life went on. One afternoon, my boss, Gary, came into my office to share the huge news that we had the mega-screen in Times Square the following week for advertising. "I need you to pull together a video that will really get people's attention."

"Gary, even a naked cowboy barely gets people's attention in Times Square," I said. But I was already envisioning a full-scale production with models and a hit song and maybe even an interactive twist. In my dozen years at the childcare company, we'd never done anything remotely as high profile as this. "How big of a budget do we have?"

"Well, that's the thing. We didn't budget for it, so we'll need to keep the costs down. If you can produce it in-house, that would probably be best," he said, shattering my nascent illusions of winning a Clio.

The video would play on one of the busiest blocks in the world and could easily get lost in the hustle. Instead of trying to compete with all the sizzle, I decided to go simple. We were selling childcare, and I knew that a beautiful portrait of a baby or young child could stop even the most cynical New Yorker in their tracks. So I strung together the most striking images we had of children in our centers—laughing, learning, and playing.

And at the end of the thirty-second reel, I included a single photograph of Dalia, taken when she was six months old, pushing up from her belly and staring right at the camera with a hint of a smile and eyes full of hope. I'd never included an image of any of my kids in the work my team produced. It felt too self-serving. But there was no way I was going to miss an opportunity to celebrate Dalia at this kind of scale.

The day the video played, my father and I took the train from Boston to New York. We made our way to Times Square, positioned ourselves directly across the street from the mega-screen, and watched as a twenty-nine-foot-high Dalia appeared every thirty seconds.

"She's really gorgeous, isn't she?" I asked rhetorically, snapping pictures of the video with my camera.

"What do you expect? She takes after her grandfather," my dad replied, looking through the lens of his own camera. We watched the video play about a dozen times before I asked the question I really wanted him to answer.

"She's going to be okay, right?"

Ever since I'd become afraid of flying, I called my dad before every flight and asked him to promise me I would make it to my destination intact. He always obliged. It was a ridiculous request, of course. But he always played along, telling me he checked in with the pilots that morning and promising me the flight would be fine. I found it oddly reassuring. This time, though, he didn't humor me.

"We're going to do everything we can to make sure of it," he answered equivocally. I wanted more. I wanted his promise.

But standing there in Times Square, looking up at Dalia looking out over the city, I felt in my bones that she would be okay. Her challenges would be far greater than anything I ever thought I'd be able to handle, but this wasn't about me. This was about her, a girl who crawled out of bed every single night and climbed up the eight stairs to our bedroom with her progressively weaker arms and legs and then pulled herself up to standing so she could wake us up to ask if she could sleep on our floor. If anyone would defy the odds, it would be her.

12

Horses and Hope

It's a peculiar dance to be realistic and optimistic at the same time when those two things are at odds. Things aren't likely to get better; in fact they'll get worse. But what if they could get better? Don't we need to devote our lives to trying?

Living in the present and doing everything possible to change the future might seem like an oxymoron. It was our oxymoronic reality. In the summer of 2013, when Dalia was eight years old, two things happened. She won a horseback riding award, and I stumbled on a promising drug trial for mitochondrial disease. Both were worthy of celebration.

Dalia's physical therapist asked if I'd ever heard of hippotherapy. "Hippotherapy?" I repeated with a lilt, and I could tell that any of the obvious jokes would disappoint her.

"Hippotherapy is therapeutic horseback riding. It can help with coordination, balance, and strength," she explained. "It might be really good for Dalia, and I think she'd enjoy it."

"She'd love that," I said, already googling "hippotherapy near me" on my phone.

Of our three kids, Dalia was always the most adventurous. When we went to Niagara Falls, she was the only one who would ride the Maid of the Mist with me into the base of the falls. Ice-cold water stung our faces as we made each turn. When it was over, Dalia asked, "Ga?" On walks, she demanded that everyone take a turn running with her wheelchair. It was most fun, apparently, when we veered her dangerously close to the boys on their skateboards. At Six Flags, she wanted to go on every roller coaster multiple times. I rode next to her, enveloping her with both my arms and legs to stabilize her around turns, keeping my eyes squeezed shut. She waved her arms overhead, eyes wide open.

I don't think it was only bravery that made Dalia a thrill seeker. It was also a way for her to move unencumbered, sailing through the falls or flying along the roller-coaster tracks, wind in her face, hair drifting behind her, and not reliant on legs that wouldn't do what she wanted them to. Horseback riding might give her that same sense of freedom, ease, and power.

The next week, I drove Dalia and Theo to a stable forty-five minutes from our home to observe a lesson.

After watching for about fifteen minutes, Dalia was ready to ride.

"My turn!" she said. From then on, we went to the stable every Saturday morning. Dalia was paired with a horse named Lexie. Theo brought her carrots and Dalia brushed her coat, and then Theo and I watched as Dalia and Lexie circled the ring. Every time they passed, Dalia beamed as she took one hand off the pommel to wave.

What must it have felt like for her to guide a half-ton animal around the inside of the barn? Why wasn't she even a little bit afraid? When I went horseback riding with the boys on a vacation in Arizona, I wanted to cry as soon as the horse started moving. I was petrified going down the small hills and somewhat shocked they let anybody who signed a waiver go out on the trail. I was sure we'd galloped for the entire ride until I saw the video afterward and realized we were barely trotting.

At the end of the summer, the stable held an awards show for all the riders. Instructors helped kids with leg braces and kids in wheelchairs and kids who just needed an arm to lean on get situated on the horses. Then the kids were led around the ring.

And Dalia got her award. She'd been to countless soccer and baseball games to watch Jonah and Theo. She'd seen them test for belts in tae kwon do. This was the first time we were all there to cheer her on. I couldn't have been any prouder if Lexie had jumped over a fence with Dalia standing on one foot and spinning a plate overhead.

—»«—

I was still basking in the afterglow when I arrived at work the next day, thinking about how Dalia wanted to sleep with her award and how Jonah and Theo proudly recounted the entire event to Rob's parents. I ate lunch at my desk and took a quick break to look for research trials. I'd been doing the same search every day for years.

Then something new came up, and I thought I misunderstood.

I ran into my friend Ilene's office with my laptop. "Read this," I urged, shoving my computer in front of her. "Oh my God," Ilene said, quickly reading the page out loud.

> EPI-743 is a new drug that is based on vitamin E. Tests have shown that it can help improve the function of cells with mitochondrial problems. It may be able to treat people with genetic disorders that affect metabolism and mitochondria.

"You need to get Dalia into this."

"I know! But how?" I was too excited to think clearly.

Ilene read the list of the doctors and scientists associated with the trial while I paced around her office. "Okay, here's a doctor who works at Stanford. We're sending him an email."

By the end of the day, the researcher called me. I'd been trying for three years to find a drug trial for Dalia, and in one afternoon I not only found one, but was on the phone with the person conducting the study. It seemed like a miracle.

Rob and I tried to contain our hopes. We still needed to formally apply and be accepted into the study. But it was impossible to curb our enthusiasm. I spent so much of my life, even pre-diagnosis and pre-kids, imagining the worst-case scenario—the plane would go down or the headache would turn out to be a brain tumor or I'd forget to unplug my flat iron and burn down the house. This time I wanted to imagine the best case.

I lay in bed at night and imagined we'd be accepted into the study and Dalia would be miraculously cured. That all this would end up being a nightmarish chapter in her story, instead of the story itself, an incredible tale we'd tell at her wedding.

Within a few weeks, I had an interview with someone from the National Human Genome Research Institute.

"To be admitted to the study we'll need documentation of a symptom that can be objectively measured and tracked, something that's declined over time and can be clinically assessed to see whether the drug makes a difference."

"What about her hearing loss?" I asked, suddenly grateful for her hearing loss.

"Absolutely, that will work for us," she said. "I'm going to need a complete copy of Dalia's medical history, and if she meets our extended list of criteria, we'll need a skin biopsy. The cells from the biopsy will be treated with the drug, and if they respond positively, and if at that point there are spaces available in the study, Dalia will be invited to participate. We should have an answer for you in about six months."

There were a whole lot of "ifs" thrown out in the conversation, and it was decidedly different from the fantasy, which had us traveling to Washington, DC, the next week. But I also felt like we were finally moving forward, even if not quite at the pace I'd have preferred.

A few months later we received an email from the National Institutes of Health (NIH):

> Her cells grew adequately and were put in the
> queue to be tested for infection in the next

> 1–2 weeks! This is great news! As long as her cells are negative for infection, we will ship to the lab with the next batch to be tested. Once at the lab it takes 2–6 weeks for them to assess. So, best case 4–8 weeks! And if she is positive, we'll find a time when you can discuss entry into the study and arrange for travel. I know this process is very long, but we're getting closer every day!

Surely there wouldn't have been four exclamation points in the email if we were meant to be cautious.

That night my dad came over to celebrate. He brought half of Whole Foods, a few bottles of wine, a bouquet of dahlias, and a bursting folder stuffed with everything he'd printed off about mitochondrial research in general and EPI-743 in particular. "You did it," he said, proudly. "Tell me if you want me to come to DC with you or stay home with the boys so you and Rob can both bring Dalia. Whatever you need." All optimism; no hesitation. "To health!" he toasted.

"To health," I replied, knocking on the kitchen table for good luck.

13

State of Emergency

We went to Florida during February school vacation. There was so much we wanted to vacate. We found an all-inclusive resort with a gigantic slide right on the beach, and off we went for cornhole on the beach, a dolphin cruise, and way too many milkshakes.

We'd escaped a bitter-cold Boston winter. The region was stuck in a polar vortex of some sort, which sounds like a sci-fi plot, but really just means it was the kind of cold that hurts your eyeballs and makes your teeth freeze. Along with their bathing suits and sun hats, the kids brought a nasty winter bug with them.

Our suite had two bedrooms, one for the boys and one for Rob, Dalia, and me. None of us was getting much sleep. The boys were staying up until sunrise watching movies, which Rob and I were ignoring out of respect for the vacation. We weren't faring nearly as well in our bedroom, where Dalia's cough and congested breathing kept all three of us awake most of the night.

For the first few days we rallied through the exhaustion, napping by the pool and, later in the day, on the beach. Theo and Jonah collected seashells while Dalia slept beside me. One evening Theo showed me how he arranged the shells on a table in his room. He'd placed a large shell and a medium one on either side of a small pink shell.

"This is Jonah, and this is me," he said, pointing to the outer shells. "The one in the middle is Dalia. The Jonah shell and the Theo shell are protecting the Dalia shell. That's our job, right, Mommy? We protect Dalia." I took him in my arms. "Yes, sweetie, we protect Dalia. And you and Jonah are the best protectors in the world."

The next morning, Dalia's bed was empty. When I reached for Rob and realized he wasn't there either, I assumed he took Dalia on an early-morning walk or the two of them were sacked out in the living room watching TV. I got out of bed still bleary-eyed and found them on the living room couch. They were disheveled and pasty despite the hint of sunburn.

Dalia was in Rob's arms, eyes glazed, half asleep, but making so much noise breathing in and out that I couldn't quite believe the boys and I—or even the people in the room next door—slept through it. She sounded like a washing machine.

I didn't want to overreact but decided to check in with Dalia's pediatrician back home so he could tell me if we should put her in a steamy bathroom, like we did when Jonah had croup and sounded like a barking seal, or whether we needed to get her some meds.

"I'm sure it's just a bad cold," the pediatrician said. But when I held the phone up to Dalia's rumbling, he changed direction. "I think it makes sense to go to an emergency room. She might need an antibiotic."

I hung up and turned to Rob. "Do you really think we need to take her?"

"I don't know," he said. "Maybe we should wait another day and see if she gets a bit better." But Dalia's labored crackling interrupted our deliberating. "Do you want to take her, or should I?" Rob asked.

"I'll go," I volunteered. "We'll meet you at the pool when we get back. Save some seats."

My limited experience with emergency rooms involved a lot of waiting. I considered that a plus, since the people bumped to the front of the line were the ones who had the least time to waste. I was always certain I'd contract something way worse than what brought me in the first place—the Zika virus or Ebola, for example—by the time they called my name.

But this time we were taken into an exam room immediately. Two nurses met us and took Dalia's vitals—heart rate, blood pressure, temperature. Then they put a little clamp on her finger to measure her oxygen and saw that it was in the low nineties, well below where it should be. They picked up their pace. "We're going to need to get her oxygen up," one nurse told me as she put a small oxygen mask over Dalia's nose and mouth. Dalia promptly took the mask off, so the nurse put two little tubes in Dalia's nostrils instead.

Dalia was half asleep, yet she managed to pull out the tubes. It was back to the mask. Then she swatted off the mask, so we tried the tubes again. We kept playing this game while more people—nurses, techs, doctors—came in and out.

I was still waiting for someone to give us the antibiotics and wondering whether we'd make it back to the hotel for lunch.

Then a new doctor came in and introduced himself.

"We're going to send you to a bigger hospital in town," he said. "St. Pete's has a pediatric ward, and they'll be able to give you more specialized care."

Within minutes, Dalia and I were in an ambulance. I sat next to the stretcher, holding one of Dalia's hands with both of mine. "We're just going to a different building to see some doctors who can give us medicine to make you all better," I promised.

But I was also somewhere else watching Dalia and me in the ambulance. I was fast-forwarding to being back at the hotel telling Rob about the ambulance ride and how I was kind of disappointed that the driver didn't turn on the siren. I was on the phone with my dad asking him to promise me my daughter was going to be okay. I was back at work telling Ilene about what a non-vacation my vacation turned out to be.

We arrived at the hospital and went through a second intake, recounting what led us to the hospital that morning and explaining about Dalia's MERRF syndrome.

The doctor gave Dalia a quick exam and then turned to me. "After your daughter is admitted, we'll run some tests and get chest X-rays." My stomach began burning as it became clear we were not making it out of the hospital with just an antibiotic prescription.

At that point Rob and I decided to swap places. We knew our respective strengths. If there was advocating, organizing, or planning to be done, I was your woman. But calm in a storm was Rob's specialty.

Later, over chicken sandwiches and fries, I did my best to hide my rising panic, to reassure the boys that Dalia and Rob would be back early the next day. We took a walk on the beach and went back to the room early for a movie. I just wanted to get to sleep, put an end to this dreadful day, reunite the family, and get back to our vacation.

It turns out that anxiety-filled surreal night was the most peaceful one I'd have for months to come. I had been told by a mitochondrial specialist just months before that people with mitochondrial disease can turn on a dime—that what's a run-of-the-mill nasty flu or even a simple cold for otherwise healthy people can be devastating for people with compromised mitochondria. But I wasn't thinking about that then. Other than the not-so-small matter of having MERRF syndrome, Dalia had been fairly healthy over the last few years. I thought our vacation would resume and we'd have one of those "remember when" stories that all families have.

The next morning Rob called. "Sweetyheart, they moved Dalia to the ICU."

"Wait, what?"

"It's okay," he said. "They just want to watch her more closely." He was doing for me exactly what I'd been doing for the boys the night before.

But an hour later, he called again and told me that Dalia aspirated on her regular morning medications, meaning instead of swallowing them, she'd inhaled them into her lungs. This time, he wasn't quite so calm.

"Her oxygen dropped so low, they needed to intubate her. It all happened so quickly, and now she has a breathing tube and she's completely sedated. There are like fifteen people in the room here right now."

I could see the boys splashing in the pool, doing a decent job of vacationing despite the curveball they'd been thrown. I tried to gauge whether I should rush them out of the pool and get us all to the hospital or try to stay calm and minimize what was going on so I wouldn't totally freak them out.

I called the pediatrician.

"Intubation is very, very serious," he began. "I think you should all get to the hospital right away and spend time together as a family." *Spend time together as a family?* This was not the time and the hospital was not the place to be together as a family. If the situation was as dire as he was suggesting, I didn't want the boys to witness it. I wanted them to think about Dalia as she was two days before, snuggled in her purple poncho on the dolphin cruise. I hung up with the doctor and called someone I knew nearby to come watch the boys so I could get to Dalia and Rob.

I ran to the front of the hotel to catch a cab to the hospital. I ran across the hospital lobby to the elevator bank. I ran from the elevator to the room number I scribbled on my hand when I was talking to Rob. And then I stopped short.

When I left Dalia at the hospital the day before, she looked weak and a bit peaked. There'd been an IV inserted in her arm, and we'd been going back and forth between the oxygen mask and the nasal cannula. (I'd never heard of a nasal cannula before, but it's now a term I toss around as lightly as "pulmonary toilet" and "mucus plug.")

Now there was a long strip of white tape that ran from one side of her face to the other, under her nose and over her mouth, covering the wires that attached to the breathing tube. She had multiple tubes coming out of each arm; I didn't know for what. There were several round stickers holding wires to her chest to monitor her heart, oxygen, and respiratory rates, and her legs were raised on a pillow with a huge piece of yellow foam encircling each of her ankles. Along each side of her bed were various machines and monitors, and behind the bed was a long strip with dozens more. She was heavily sedated, wearing an impossibly cheerful hospital gown, with her brown stuffed doggie lying across her body.

Rob came to the door of the room, and I collapsed into his arms for a few seconds. Then I took a deep breath, trying to calm my racing heart, and went over to the bed. I was so afraid to touch Dalia. I didn't want to dislodge a tube or a wire or set off an alarm. I tentatively reached out my hand and began stroking her forehead, just the way she liked it.

A few minutes later, the doctor came to meet us.

"I'm Dr. Meyers. Dalia's stable, we're taking good care of her. We have her oxygen up, and she's finally getting the sleep she's clearly needed. I've been reading up on MERRF syndrome. This is a new one for me. Can you tell me how it presents in Dalia?"

I started with the hearing loss, and when I got to the word "ataxia," she interrupted me.

"Can you hold on a second?" She stepped out of the room and came back with another doctor and two nurses. A respiratory therapist and a social worker followed. "Do you mind starting again from the beginning?" Suddenly I was giving a mini-seminar on MERRF syndrome.

I didn't want to be the teacher. I didn't know enough, was afraid I'd say something misleading or factually incorrect. I heard myself explaining what I knew, trying to sound competent. But I could feel the adrenaline coursing through my body as I realized we knew more than the people we were counting on to heal our daughter. I wanted to ask to speak to the manager, the person in charge, the doctor who could wave a magic wand and make Dalia all better.

─ »《 ─

Dalia's aspiration caused pneumonia, and after three days in the hospital she wasn't getting any better. We couldn't keep up the facade for the boys any longer, so I called Rachel and asked her to fly out, get the boys, and bring them home.

Rob and I checked out of the hotel and into Dalia's hospital room. The room was beautiful, with windows that overlooked the ocean, a full-size pullout couch, and a private bathroom. In this gorgeous space, Dalia remained intubated with all kinds of tubes going into and coming out of her body. She didn't panic or cry or complain, but I did. The strength of Dalia's spirit compensated for her fragile little body.

We sat vigil by her bed, waiting for any sign that she was getting better. We tried to sleep while she slept, just like when she was a baby. But the noise and the panic and the steady stream of people kept us up most of the night.

We waited for the doctors to give us a morsel of good news—even a hint that Dalia was getting stronger. We waited for the sun to rise so we could have another day that might bring some improvement. We waited for the sun to set so we could try to get some rest. And then, after five days of waiting, Dr. Meyers arrived before sunrise.

"I have good news. I think Dalia's ready to be extubated, so I've put orders in. We'll take out the breathing tube this afternoon and let Dalia breathe on her own."

"Oh, thank God," I said, standing. Our vigil was over—we could pack our bags and put this whole episode behind us. My shoulders, which had been tightly lodged next to my ears all week, began to drop.

14

Strings

There was just one catch.

The doctor explained that after the extubation Dalia would need to be closely monitored in the hospital until she regained her strength.

"How long will that be?" Rob asked.

Please say a few days. Please say a few days.

"No way to know," Dr. Meyers said. "It could be as little as a couple of weeks, but it could take longer, especially if she needs to go to rehab before returning home."

"That's impossible," I said. "We have two other kids. We can't just stay here indefinitely."

"Well, there is one other option," she offered. "You could fly home while Dalia is intubated. With the breathing tube in place, the ventilator will keep her safer than her lungs can right now."

"I'll call the airline now," I said, pivoting to grab my phone.

Of course that was what we'd do. We could be home in just a few hours.

"Wait, Jessica. It's not that simple," she said. I stopped short, my body still facing away.

"You'll need to fly home on a medical jet, and that needs to go through insurance."

It didn't occur to me that you can't simply board Jet-Blue while intubated. An air ambulance was all we'd need, and apparently we were in luck because we could rent one for $30,000 if the insurance company didn't agree to foot the bill. Our choices were to take out the breathing tube and stay in Florida for what would be an indefinite recovery period or convince the insurance company to cover our flight. A twisted version of *Let's Make a Deal*.

But wait, there was more. The doctor told us we had just twenty-four hours to decide whether we were going to take out the breathing tube in Florida or fly home with Dalia intubated. Each day of intubation comes with risk, so now that Dalia was strong enough to breathe on her own, we couldn't let the inconvenience of being in Florida cause a delay.

Within the hour, a social worker came to talk to us. She assured us the insurance request for a medical transfer would be approved, told us she'd never had a family be denied when there was a medical necessity for it.

"But there is one thing," she said. "There's a decent chance the insurance company will only approve a flight to Atlanta. We've connected with a mitochondrial specialist there, and since Atlanta is considerably closer to Florida than Boston is, it would be a less expensive flight."

We were getting used to the "catches," the "buts," the "one things," but the notion that we'd relocate to Atlanta seemed like a particularly cruel twist. Surely the insurance company wouldn't keep us from our family to save a few dollars on gas.

The social worker gave me a quick arm hug, told us to "sit tight," and said she'd let us know just as soon as she heard anything.

Sitting tight is not my forte. No matter how determined and competent this social worker was—and I had no way at that point to assess either one of those things—getting us back to Boston was likely not even in the top five most important things on her to-do list that day. Getting us back to Boston was the only thing on my list.

The alternative to Boston, whether it was Florida or Atlanta, was impossible. *What would that even look like? Would we rent an apartment near the hospital and move the boys out to be with us? Would I ask Rachel to take care of the boys indefinitely? And what about our jobs?*

I called insurance directly, but I couldn't figure out which of the recorded options applied to us. Apparently the people who work the phones to update claim statuses or replace lost cards aren't the same ones responsible for making $30,000 decisions. I called my family and friends who'd been living the play-by-play with me since we were admitted to the hospital, begging for reassurance that it was going to be okay.

When the social worker came back to our room, she started with the arm hug.

"We were denied," she said softly. "I'm going to appeal, but we don't have much time. I'm so sorry. I really didn't expect this to happen."

I didn't want her apology, had no time to appease her. The arm hugs were just annoying. I knew we needed to take control of the situation, though I didn't really know how to do that. I grabbed my phone and ran into the hall, where there was better reception. Who did I know who might know someone at the insurance company? I was ready to pull any strings I could find, no matter how flimsy. While I was doing that, Rob was trying to figure out if we could pull together $30,000 to pay for the flight ourselves. Could we ask six people to give us $5,000 each? Fifteen people for $2,000?

I called my father and my sister, and then I called my friend Kara. She and her family were exceedingly well connected, the kind of people who know someone who can get you a passport thirty-six hours before your overseas flight when you realize yours is expired (yes, that happened) or call their contacts in the Guatemalan government when your adoption case is tied up in endless spools of red tape (that happened too). Sure enough, Kara's brother was friends with someone senior at the insurance company. While all this sounds a bit pat and somewhat questionable—maybe even a bit mob-like—it was all aboveboard. Which isn't to suggest that I wouldn't have called in connections that weren't aboveboard if I thought they could help us get home.

I've been known to have incredibly bad luck. When people say "one in a million," I'm the one. When we were bringing Dalia home from Guatemala, our plane was struck by lightning. On a flight from Boston to Los Angeles, the guy in the seat next to me died. Literally. (Apparently, he had worse luck than I do.) I had chicken pox three times. In college, my roommates and I returned from spring break to learn that one of the apartments in our massive student housing complex had been destroyed by burst pipes. Yep, ours. And there were bigger, more life-altering things too. All those years of bad luck trying to get pregnant, for example.

Now I felt like I was being repaid in some cosmic way for all the bad luck I'd experienced to that point. What are the chances that Kara knew somebody at the insurance company we needed to get on our side? Even less than one in a million.

I quickly crafted an email explaining our situation, trying to strike the right balance between rationality and heart-string tugging.

What I wrote:

> I am writing about my daughter, Dalia, who suffers from MERRF syndrome, a rare mito-chondrial disease. Dalia's disease is debili-tating in many ways, including an inability to walk, hearing loss, muscle weakness, etc. Last week we traveled from Boston to St. Petersburg, Florida, for vacation. On Wednes-day she became ill, and we took her to the ER. She was transferred to All Children's Hospital in St. Petersburg and admitted. Shortly there-after they moved her to the ICU. She aspirated and was then intubated. She has been intu-bated since Thursday.

The doctors here at All Children's have submitted a request with Air Ambulance to transfer Dalia to Mass General Hospital, so she can be cared for by her team of physicians. There is no mitochondrial specialist at the Florida hospital or in the vicinity. All of the doctors involved agree that it would be much safer to transfer Dalia while intubated than shortly after extubation. It is unclear how long her recovery will be once she is extubated. Obviously, time is of the essence with this request.

Please let me know if I can provide any additional information. Thank you.

What I didn't write:

For the past week I've been petrified that my daughter is going to die. She's been so brave; so much braver than I have. I'm scared these doctors don't understand her disease the way her doctors in Boston do. I also have two little boys who are living with my sister right now. They're sad and confused. She bought them five new LEGO sets and has been giving them ice cream for breakfast every day to try to distract them, but they just want to see their sister. Please just be a good person and fly us home.

We were in some strange time warp where the hours were both crawling and flying by. I felt a new urgency to be on our home turf, and every minute we remained in limbo was a personal insult. At the same time, I willed the clock to slow. I wanted as much time as possible to let the appeals team ponder our case. We were dealing with the social worker and the phone calls and the emails, and we were focused on what was happening to Dalia—on grabbing every second we could with the doctors, on pleading with the nurses and the various therapists who came in and out to give us some ray of hope, on holding Dalia's hand and trying to distract her with stories and silly songs.

At 10:30 the next morning, the social worker came by to tell us the appeal was denied—she didn't even bother with the arm hug this time.

I'd been perfectly obsequious up to that point, trying to get on her good side so she might put in an extra bit of effort, but now the mama bear within started to growl.

I felt my whole body tighten as I heard myself say, "What do you mean it's been denied?" I was desperate. "Can't they at least fly us to Atlanta? We'll take Atlanta! How can we change their minds?"

She stood silent. Rob was outside of our conversation focusing on Dalia, while I stopped just short of calling the social worker an incompetent boob.

My rant was interrupted by my ringing phone, and I glanced down and saw it was the insurance company.

I fumbled, "Hello?"

"I'm happy to tell you your request for a flight transfer home has been approved," the person who was apparently the Messiah said. "We've arranged for a flight first thing tomorrow morning." I thanked her profusely, hung up the phone, and told the social worker I believed she was mistaken, that we had in fact been approved.

I knew the only reason we were able to go home was because a friend of a friend moved our request to the top of the pile or put in an urgent word for us. I felt guilty about that, wondering about the family in the room next to ours or on the floor above who might not be so lucky. I couldn't understand how what felt like a life-or-death decision came down to connections. Insurance was supposed to be our safety net, but if not for our friend, it would have let us fall. Those thoughts were fleeting though, because I had calls to make, family to update, bags to pack.

My fear of flying evaporated. On a tiny plane with no bathroom, my daughter sedated on a stretcher beside me, with all the turbulence you'd expect in the middle of winter, the only thing I worried about was Dalia. In just a few hours we were back at our home hospital. Back to a world we hoped would feel less Kafkaesque and more like a fairy tale in which we could wake up from this nightmare and live happily ever after.

15

Life in the PICU

The pediatric intensive care unit (PICU) is separate from the time and space that gives order to our lives. It's eerily quiet and deafeningly loud at the same time—with people talking in hushed voices amid the cacophony of beeps and alarms that never stop. The rooms are dim during the day, but the lights are turned on and off throughout the night as numbers are recorded, medication is administered, and vitals are checked. ICU psychosis is a real thing, and it didn't take long to understand why.

The doctors in the PICU at Mass General met Dalia when she was intubated, battling pneumonia, and weakened from her hospital stay in Florida. Having no basis for comparison and knowing she had mitochondrial disease, they assumed she was more symptomatic and weaker than she actually was. They asked who her pulmonologist was. I asked what a pulmonologist was. They asked how frequently she had grand mal seizures. I told them she'd never had a grand mal seizure. I explained to each new person on the case that the day before she was intubated, she had been happily eating chicken nuggets and potato chips poolside with her brothers.

After a week of trying to paint a picture of her life before, I hung a few photos of Dalia on the wall so they could get a sense of who she was. I thought that if they saw the pictures of her sunbathing on a lounge chair, leading a presentation on Guatemala to her fellow third graders, or blowing out her birthday candles the year before, they'd be more committed to getting her through this and making sure she emerged as feisty and gregarious as ever. I wanted them to see that despite her diagnosis of MERRF syndrome, she was not a sick kid.

As one week in the Mass General PICU became two, our world started to shrink. Being with Dalia and taking care of our boys was all that mattered. Just a month earlier Rob and I were consumed with our jobs. Like most of our friends, we spent the majority of our waking hours at work, with family responsibilities crammed into the periphery. But now we had neither the time nor the inclination to spend any mental or emotional energy on anything beyond our children. Work wasn't a welcome distraction; it was an impossible one. Rob and I both took leaves of absence from work.

It wasn't lost on us how lucky we were to have employers who supported us through this crisis. We knew there were others in the PICU who had to leave their kids in the morning to go to work and return just in time to say good night. We saw them leave in their work clothes; we saw them hurry back in the evening. For the most part, the doors all along the hallway were open throughout the day, and we got a sense of what was going on inside each room. We walked by our neighbors on our way in and out of the unit, always averting our eyes to give them an illusion of privacy, just as we wanted them to do when they passed our room. But we couldn't help but hear the young children crying, the loud moans of the older kids.

We didn't get to know any of the other parents. There was no bonding over shared circumstance or late nights comparing notes about the nurses. The most we offered each other was a feeble smile while we waited by the elevator or in line for the bathroom. We were all consumed by our own tragedies, sinking in our particular quicksand. We didn't have the strength to reach out to the strangers sinking beside us. Maybe we didn't want to see them go under for fear we'd meet the same fate. Maybe we didn't want to watch them escape while we were still descending.

Rob and I quickly settled into a rhythm—albeit a somewhat discordant one—in which one of us spent the night at the hospital while the other ate dinner with the boys and slept at home. I hated the nights I was at the hospital, trying to comfort Dalia, missing the boys, unable to sleep. I hated the nights I wasn't at the hospital, trying to comfort the boys, missing Dalia, unable to sleep. In the morning, the one of us who was home got the boys off to school and then raced to the hospital. When I spent the night at the hospital, I counted the minutes in the morning until Rob returned. Being there alone was alternately scary and boring, and always depleting.

You don't get much sleep in the PICU. You want to wear earplugs to drown out the incessant beeps, but you don't dare do it for fear you won't be able to hear when your daughter whispers your name or slaps the bed to get your attention when the breathing tube prevents her from uttering even a whisper. You bring pillows and a comforter from home when it's clear this will be more than a weekend stay, but short of bringing a pillow-top mattress, you can't mask the fact that you're sleeping on an unforgiving vinyl couch. Your back knows better. You dread when the nurses come in, because they're going to suction or take vitals or reposition your daughter, any one of which will wake her up. You are desperate for her to sleep, which is one of the only things that's going to help her get strong enough to get out of the hospital. But you also wish the nurses would come in more frequently. You crave their expertise and reassurance.

It's somewhat surprising that life in the PICU is as boring as it is. I once read a description of war that said it was days of boredom punctuated by brief periods of bloody and terrifying action. Same with the PICU.

Of course, given the choice, we'd all choose monotony every time. But the monotony is just so, well, monotonous.

You spend most of the day waiting—waiting for doctors to make their rounds, waiting for someone to arrive who can guard your post so you can leave the room to go to the bathroom, waiting for even the slightest indication that your daughter is starting to get better. You wait for medicine to kick in when your daughter is in pain, and you wait for medicine to wear off so she can be alert and communicative.

The tedium is broken by episodes of intense anxiety that come crashing on top of the normal anxiety that's there all the time. The nature of the PICU is that every patient is in a dire situation. It's inevitable that tragedy strikes, that you hear the alarms going off, that you see the full on-duty staff rush into a patient's room. When that happens, you hold your daughter's hand and try to distract her. You pull out an art project or sing her a song and silently pray that your neighbor is going to make it. You feel so relieved when it's another room, not yours. You feel so bad for feeling so good.

Once in a while the code alarms go off in your room. Your daughter is the patient that the doctors are urgently surrounding. You still hold her hand and try to distract her, but the doctors gently push you aside so they can do their job. Your silent prayers are more urgent now. You bargain with a god you're not sure you believe in. You promise to be a better parent, a better person, a better human being. You're not sure you know what any of that means, but you promise to figure it out.

16

Longing for Boredom

The ups and downs in the PICU made the roller coaster of fertility treatments seem like a merry-go-round. A few days after we returned to Boston, Dalia's breathing tube was going to be removed. The procedure was scheduled for 11:00 a.m., and my plan was to head to the hospital as soon as I got the boys off to school. This was what we'd been waiting for, the step that would get us one step closer to bringing Dalia home. With the breathing tube out, Dalia would be able to talk. I was desperate to hear her voice again. All this time I'd been telling her she'd be okay; I wanted to hear her reassure me that she was.

I'd just walked Theo to the bus stop when Rob called.

"They moved up the procedure," he said. "They're doing it in a few minutes."

"Tell them to wait! I'm on my way," I said, hoping my schedule might take precedence over the doctors'.

Forty-five minutes later, I was sitting in my Subaru on the Mass Pike screaming at the cars that were crawling in front of me when my phone dinged. I glanced down and saw that Rob sent me a video. I hit "play," instantly grateful that the traffic was at a virtual standstill. There, on my screen, was Dalia.

"Hi, Mama," she said in her high-pitched lilt, her smile taking up half of her face. "I miss you. I wuv you." That was it, and it was all I needed. I must have watched that video three hundred times and sent it to almost everyone I'd ever met. I was prouder of her at that moment than I'd been when she said her very first word seven or so years earlier.

I called Rob. "How does she seem? Does her throat hurt? Did they say anything about when she'll be able to come home?" I pummeled him with questions. "Make a list, and we can ask the doctor everything during rounds," he said. "On it!" I said. Any excuse to make a list was good with me.

We were giddy, daring to hope we were nearing the end of the horrible saga. We thought we'd go home a bit worse for wear, more cautious about traveling in the future, and more hypervigilant at the first sign of a cold.

But Dalia's lungs kept getting weaker. Her low oxygen set off alarms, and her lungs needed to be suctioned over and over. Every time we heard fluid crackling in her little body, I raced out to the nurse's station.

"She needs suctioning! She's making noise!" I shouted at anyone who looked official. They took their time. Of all the things that were happening in the PICU, this was clearly not the most serious.

That should have reassured me, I suppose. But I was braced for impact.

Two nights after Dalia's breathing tube was taken out, my friend Karen came to sit with me in the hospital. I was rubbing Dalia's forehead.

"My shoulders are killing me," I moaned, taking the hand that wasn't caressing Dalia and contorting myself to knead my own shoulder.

"Here, let me give you a back rub," Karen offered.

We looked like the massage train my friends and I used to make at camp, each of us rubbing the shoulders of the person in front of us.

Karen dug into my knots, and it was as though she'd opened a spigot that had been rusted shut for years. My fear poured out.

"I'm so scared," I whispered, not wanting Dalia to hear me. "I seriously feel like I might throw up. What if something happens tonight when I'm here alone? What if she doesn't get better? What if she gets worse?"

"Of course you feel all those things. The only thing you can do is try to focus on this moment. She's okay right now. Look, she's falling asleep. Let's try to breathe together."

So we did. We took deep breaths. Karen gave me an Ativan. And Dalia and I both slept soundly.

Two nights later I was woken from my ICU semi-slumber by the sound of a small vacuum. I opened my eyes and saw several people surrounding Dalia's bed. I recognized one of the night nurses, Wendy, but didn't know the others.

One person was suctioning mucus from Dalia's lungs via a tube that went in through her nose and down the back of her throat. She paused only to let someone else draw blood.

"What's happening?" I shouted, trying to make myself heard over the din of the machines. I tried to squeeze through the people so I could hold Dalia, but I couldn't get close enough.

"Dalia's desatting," Wendy said. "We're trying to get her oxygen up." I looked at the screen near Dalia's bed that showed her oxygen level and her heart rate. I now knew what the numbers meant, and I could see her heart rate was elevated and her oxygen saturation was too low. "We're going to test her blood gas and find out if she's going into respiratory failure," Wendy said, pausing to give me the requisite arm hug.

Through it all, Dalia remained sound asleep, which I was grateful for but also really scared me because it was evidence of just how weak she'd become.

After they suctioned Dalia's lungs and took her blood and poked and prodded her little body, everyone left the room. I pulled a chair over to Dalia's bed and rested my head on the pillow beside her. A few minutes passed, and a young doctor came into the room and introduced herself.

"Mind if I sit with you for a bit?" she asked.

She looked so young, like Doogie Howser if Doogie Howser were female and Indian.

"Sure," I said, but only because I didn't think I had a choice. I preferred to sit quietly with Dalia.

"I'm glad to meet you," she began, "though I wish it were under different circumstances. I've heard a lot about your daughter. She sounds like quite a little fighter."

It didn't surprise me that she'd heard about Dalia. I knew the doctors on call read the charts of each patient in the PICU, but also Dalia's reputation always preceded her.

"She is amazing," I agreed.

"How are you doing?" she asked.

"It all feels surreal," I began. "I don't know how we got here, and I don't know when we're going to get out. I don't know how to make Dalia better."

"Dalia's going to tell us what she needs," she said.

"Dalia has no idea what she needs. None of us does," I said, half asleep and fully confused.

"Her body will tell us. Medicine is equal parts art and science, but we're going to listen to Dalia's symptoms. She'll tell us if she needs more oxygen. If her lungs aren't doing what they need to, then we're going to help them along."

I nodded and looked back at Dalia's face. Her long lashes didn't flutter.

The notion that Dalia would tell us what she needed—that it wasn't on Rob and me to figure out—felt like a huge relief. All along we'd been twisting ourselves in knots with each decision that was made, from titrating medication to adjusting ventilator settings, wondering how much of it all was a guessing game. That somehow Dalia was dictating what she needed, that in a way she was in charge, lifted a weight I hadn't realized had been crushing me.

Before long, Doogie's pager beeped. "The results are here," she said, unclasping the beeper from her jacket. "I'll be back in a minute."

I clutched Dalia's hand and worked on my breathing. Three seconds in; three seconds out. "Please God, please God, please God," I said in time to each breath I took.

The doctor rushed back in just a few deep breaths later. "I'm afraid it's not good news," she blurted. "We need to intubate Dalia right away."

The room started spinning.

"You need to wait in the family room," nurse Wendy, who suddenly materialized, told me. Doctors and nurses were rushing in with carts overflowing with equipment. "I want to stay," I urged. "I need to be with her." But nobody was listening. They didn't care what I needed. They knew what Dalia didn't need: a semi-hysterical mother taking up space in the room that was now bursting with people.

I stood outside the room and I didn't call Rob, because it was the middle of the night and why have both of us be totally exhausted the next day? Instead, I called my cousin Karen, who rarely slept, and together we silently waited.

Thirty minutes later, my new friend the young doctor came to tell me that all had gone well. Dalia was intubated, sedated, and stable. I made my way back to the room, lay on my "bed," and cried until morning.

–»«–

Over the next few months Dalia was intubated and extubated three times each, sometimes on my watch and sometimes on Rob's. Each intubation was dramatic and terrifying. The extubations, too, were terrifying, but they were cloaked in so much hope we didn't notice the fear quite as much.

That was life in the PICU—hating the boredom but relishing it, too, because boredom means things are copacetic. Boredom means nobody's rushing into your room. Boredom means you've made it through another day or, sometimes even more important, another night.

One morning, four weeks later, I arrived at the hospital having gotten the boys off to school and completed my battle with Boston rush hour. At that time of day, the main lobby of Mass General was like a crowded train station. People rushed in all directions dressed in every emotion you can imagine. I saw doctors and nurses striding purposefully into the building while their colleagues who worked the night shift left drained and disheveled. There was a waddling woman who looked like she might give birth right there in the lobby shuffling by a middle-aged man pushing his father in a wheelchair. I spotted two women sobbing in the corner and quickly averted my eyes so as not to intrude on their despair. There was a long line snaking out of the coffee shop, affirming my last-minute decision to stop at the Dunkin' near our house. I rounded the corner on a harpsichordist. I knew her music was meant to calm, so I stopped for a minute to listen and tried to slow my breathing.

I was precariously balancing my Diet Coke and Rob's coffee and my bag of new art supplies for Dalia when I heard someone call my name.

Right there in the lobby was Dalia, flanked by Rob and our favorite nurse.

Yes, she was in a wheelchair and attached to an IV pole, but she was out of bed and out of the PICU and right there in the middle of the swarms of people. She had a huge smile on her face as she looked up at me and softly, breathily, said, "Hi, Mama." It was the first time I'd seen her out of a hospital room in thirty-six days, and it was the first hint that we might make it out of this mess.

There was an eerie familiarity to the feeling of seeing her there, of watching her come into sharp focus as the rest of the people faded to a blur. It was almost exactly like meeting her for the first time all those years ago in the lobby of the Marriott in Guatemala City. Like then, we were surrounded by intense drama and uncertainty, by families being made and people leaving forever those they loved most. Like then, we were part of that drama but apart from it. We were simply mother and daughter. Rightfully and inextricably linked. I leaned down, took her in my arms, and held her tight. Then and now.

17

A Box on a Shelf

Even when Dalia was intubated in the ICU with no signs of improvement, Rob and I didn't think of her as a sick kid. We were so mired in what was happening each day, we simply didn't consider that her disease had progressed irreversibly. It was like standing right up close to the Georges Seurat print I bought at the Museum of Modern Art years earlier. I could see all the dots clearly, the blues, the greens, the yellows. But I had to back up to see that together all those dots formed a tree and a river, a sailboat and a rower. In the hospital, we never backed up.

After six weeks in the hospital, I met a doctor I'd successfully avoided for years, who urged me to take in the whole picture.

"I recommend you consult with Dr. O'Malley," one of Dalia's doctors suggested shortly after her initial diagnosis. "She runs the palliative care program here at the hospital, and she's a good person for you to know."

"Why would we need to meet with a palliative care doctor?" I asked, horrified at the suggestion.

The doctor heard how insulted I was and tried to back-pedal. "Palliative care can be useful for people with any kind of serious illness. It provides a holistic approach to dealing with complex physical and emotional symptoms, and Pat O'Malley is amazing. I think you'd really like her."

"I'm not sure we're ready for palliative care, but I'll think about it," I said, knowing we weren't going to think about it. "Thanks for the recommendation, though."

Palliative care was for people much sicker than Dalia.

When we were admitted to Mass General, we started hearing about Pat O'Malley again.

"You might want to consider a meeting with Pat O'Malley," the medical resident suggested. "She's a fabulous person to have on your team."

"I'm not sure if you know Pat O'Malley," the social worker said. "A lot of families in the ICU find her extremely helpful."

"Of course I know Pat," Dalia's pediatrician said. "I'd follow her across a desert."

She seemed like a mythological creature, someone everyone knew and spoke about in hushed reverential tones.

My friend Lara came to be with me at the hospital every single day, so she heard about Dr. O'Malley almost as much as I did. "Jesus, Jess," she said. "Will you just meet her already so everyone will stop bugging you about it?"

Lara was right. Plus, we had endless time at the hospital, and I was running out of excuses. I finally met Pat O'Malley one afternoon in an empty exam room while Dalia and Rob were napping.

Based on her reputation, I expected chirping birds and fluttering butterflies to accompany her into the room.

"I've read Dalia's medical file," she began. "But I'd love to hear about her from you. What's she like? What are her favorite things to do?"

I realized I'd been holding my breath, worried I was going to be forced to think about things I found unthinkable. But talking about Dalia? That I could do all day long. I released my stale breath and smiled.

"My mother used to say Dalia was an old soul. Even as a baby it took a lot to ruffle her feathers. I think that's why my sister-in-law calls her the Dalia Lama. She's a girlie girl. She loves shopping and getting her nails done and having special spa days at home with me. But she also loves wrestling with her brothers. Rob picks her up and turns her into a ninja girl, spinning her around and helping her karate kick the boys. Her favorite songs are 'Danger Zone' and 'Eye of the Tiger.' When I get home from work, she rubs my back and asks me to tell her about my day. I think she's the sweetest person ever created."

I blathered on for about fifteen minutes. When I finished, Dr. O'Malley looked at me warmly and said, "She sounds like an incredible kid. When did you first suspect something was wrong?"

I filled her in on the whole saga, starting with the hearing loss and ending with the transfer from Florida back to Boston. Somehow, we weren't talking about nail polish and sibling wrestling matches anymore.

"Let's talk about some different scenarios," Dr. O'Malley said. She explained that healthy people swallow about one thousand times a day and produce a quart of saliva. But, she said, there are people who lose their ability to swallow altogether. These people ingest all their food through a feeding tube and need to have their saliva—the entire quart each day—removed by a suction machine.

Why in the world is she telling me this? And how much longer do I need to stay here?

Dr. O'Malley also wanted to talk about major decisions Rob and I might need to make—things like whether to put a "do not resuscitate" order in Dalia's file and what we'd do if Dalia's quality of life became severely compromised.

I considered putting my hands over my ears and shouting, "I'm not listening, I'm not listening," but I thought she might find that rude. I think maybe I actually did block my ears for a few seconds, because Pat jumped in and said, "Why don't we take that conversation and put it in a box. We'll stick it on a shelf in the closet, and we can take it down if we want or need to in the future."

"Please don't take this personally," I said, "but I don't think I like you very much."

"I understand," she said with a smile. "Why don't we go back to the room? I want to meet the Dalia Lama for myself."

—»«—

I called my father to debrief. "Can you believe there are people who can't swallow their own saliva?" I asked. "Doesn't that sound awful?"

"Yes, it does sound awful," he replied. "You know what else sounds awful? The fact that I have no food in my house.

How about I pick up dinner for us all and meet you back at the house around 6:00?"

We felt lucky that not being able to swallow was something totally removed from our own reality—like amputated limbs or cleft palates—something that had nothing to do with us.

Over the next several weeks, Dr. O'Malley stopped by to visit us in our hospital room a few times a week, and before long I grew to trust her more than anyone else at the hospital. She had an ethereal quality of suddenly appearing in the room when there were major decisions to be made or particularly stressful things happening, in a "you got this," reassuring way. She never appeared empty-handed. She brought purple nail polish and bubbles for Dalia or a book for me.

I hated that she brought up things I didn't want to think about, much less talk about, but I also respected that she was gently trying to prepare me for the realities we'd likely face, that she didn't let the fact that I told her outright that I didn't like her dissuade her from being my friend. She seemed all-knowing without being a know-it-all—a delicate balance she struck perfectly.

I found that first conversation with Pat wildly uncomfortable, but I loved the notion of the box on a shelf in the closet. There was so much I wanted to put in that box. Who was going to take our kids if something happened to Rob and me? Asking someone to take on three kids was a giant request. Add the fact that one of those kids has a rare disease, and it became an impossible one. Put it in the box.

Would my job be waiting for me when at long last we emerged from the hospital? Even if it was, would I be able to keep up the same pace I had before? Right in the box.

What in God's name was the hospital bill going to look like? Box.

And there was more. Were we permanently scarring Jonah and Theo with our laser focus on Dalia? In the box.

And most important, was Dalia ever going to make it home? It's surprising to me that the shelf didn't buckle altogether, given how much weight I put in that box.

"So? *Nu?*" Lara asked when she arrived the night after I first met Dr. O'Malley, handing me a turkey sandwich and Diet Coke. "What do we think of her?"

"I think we hate her, but we probably love her too," I said.

By this point Dalia was sound asleep, and Lara and I were lying together on the small hard couch across from her bed. The Academy Awards were on, and Lara had brought popcorn and Raisinets for show snacks.

"Do you want to talk about it?" Lara asked.

"Not even a little bit," I said. "Let's talk about the dresses."

Later, if I was feeling particularly emboldened, I'd take the box down. I'd lift the lid and peek inside. I might even go so far as to take one item out and consider it for a while, turn it over in my hands and see how it felt. But as soon as I started to feel anxious or uncomfortable, back in it would go. I knew the box would be waiting for me when I was ready or even demand my attention when I wasn't, but meeting with Dr.

O'Malley was enough for the day. I needed some normalcy, and watching the Academy Awards with Lara was the perfect distraction, even if we were curled up in a hospital room with Dalia's machines hissing in the background.

18

Surrender

Dalia's medical team began to press us to make a decision that was too urgent and too huge to stuff in the box.

When Dalia was intubated for the third time, the doctors urged us to agree to an operation called a tracheostomy, where they'd put a dime-size hole in Dalia's neck that would go directly into her windpipe. A tube would be inserted through the hole to help clear her airway and get more oxygen to her lungs. It would guarantee no more intubations, since the tube can attach to an external ventilator that would control Dalia's breathing. It's essentially like a permanent, on-the-go intubation. It would also put an end to all the invasive, painful suctioning of mucus and saliva through Dalia's nose and down her throat, because suctioning happens right through the trach.

What was at first a hypothetical dropped into conversation every third day or so now became a primary focus. For the most part the doctors spoke about it in academic terms. They told us about the ways a tracheostomy would help Dalia from a respiratory perspective, that it might in fact be the only way we were ever going to be able to leave the hospital.

I was horrified that the doctors would even mention it, let alone recommend it. Because while it might make sense practically as a way to fix the respiratory nightmare, the trach would likely mean Dalia wouldn't be able to speak anymore.

"I totally understand why you'd bring this up, but it's not something we're interested in," I said the first dozen or so times.

I was delirious with exhaustion, and everything in my body hurt. My jaw was tight from so much clenching. My hair hurt from keeping it in a bun every minute of the day and night. My back ached from sleeping on the pretend bed. My stomach seized from the three pounds of chocolate I ate each day. My heart throbbed from all of it.

"We're not talking about the trach," I said after my politeness ran its course.

They thought they might have better luck with Rob. One of the doctors took him into a conference room and showed him a trach. She took it out of its box and put it on the table. Rob picked it up and turned it in his hands.

"It will allow us to put air directly into her lungs, bypassing her nose and mouth," the doctor explained.

"Do we have other options?" Rob asked.

"Well, some families decide not to go with the trach. In those cases, sometimes we just make the kids as comfortable as possible, and then . . ."

"Don't ever bring that up with me again," Rob interrupted, standing and walking out of the room.

By then we had already agreed to an operation to place a gastrostomy tube (G-tube) in Dalia's belly, which is a feeding tube through which food and medication can be given, a far better alternative to the feeding tube that threaded up her nose and down into her stomach.

But weirdly enough, I knew a bit about tracheostomy-like operations, and it wasn't something I was prepared to consider for Dalia.

When I was twenty-two, my stepfather, Frank, was diagnosed with laryngeal cancer and had to have a laryngectomy, which removed his voice box and separated his airway from his mouth and nose. After the surgery, Frank carried a medical card that officially declared him a "total neck breather." He breathed through a hole in his neck, called a stoma. Without a voice box, he couldn't speak.

After Frank's surgery, I often found my mother crying alone downstairs on the living room couch. The loss of Frank's voice was her loss too. I gave her space, never letting on that I saw how much despair she was going through. I wish I'd gone and lay beside her, even once. But her sadness scared me, and I thought it best to leave it, and her, alone.

The thought that Dalia, just nine, might get a hole in her neck and lose her ability to speak was intolerable.

One morning during rounds, right in the middle of the usual rundown of stats and suggested next steps, Dr. Navinsky, one of the ICU doctors, let it slip that "having a child with a tracheostomy is a nightmare." I'd felt a particular bond with this doctor as soon as I found out he was Israeli. I tried out my rudimentary Hebrew on him, and he at least pretended to be impressed. I was always trying to bond with the doctors and specialists. I wanted them to like us and to add every bit of incremental effort to

Dalia's care. "*Shalom*, Dr. Navinsky. *Mah nishma?*" I'd say in greeting. He humored me and responded with a simple "*B'seder*," suspecting correctly that I wouldn't be able to understand much more than that.

Dr. Navinsky didn't elaborate on why exactly having a child with a trach is a nightmare, and we didn't ask. We knew where we fell on the issue, so his observation was merely further proof that we were right to resist.

Most of the other doctors, however, felt a trach was inevitable and that we were procrastinating by refusing to move forward. We continued to resist it, to insist she just needed more time. We told ourselves she was still recovering from the pneumonia, that her body was getting stronger ever so slowly. We searched for any evidence that could lend credibility to our stance. See? Today she was awake for two hours before falling back asleep. Did you hear that? She just kind of, sort of laughed.

Yet when I lay in Dalia's room at night, listening to the churn of the machines, I wrestled with the idea that her extended illness was likely not a fluke, that her body had become so weak from her underlying mitochondrial disease that it couldn't contend anymore with the germs and the bugs and the viruses and infections that for most of us are merely an inconvenience. I googled pictures of kids with trachs and studied the ones where the kids were smiling. *This kid looks happy. Could Dalia have a happy life with a trach? Could we?*

But morning came, and we returned to our list of the pros and cons of the surgery. We always got stuck on the one con that drowned out everything else. If Dalia got a tracheostomy, she would lose her ability to speak. How could we do that to her? How could we silence our child who was already becoming marginalized by her disease in so many ways? Weren't the wheelchair, hearing aids, leg braces, and feeding tube enough?

It would be one thing, I suppose, if she were in a horrible accident and was given an emergency tracheostomy to save her life. It would be another thing altogether if she were born with a condition that prevented her from ever speaking. But we weren't in either of those situations. We were being asked to voluntarily elect to have Dalia's voice removed.

Who were we to make that call? Yes, I realized, better us— her parents—than anyone else. But we were in so deep over our heads. We couldn't begin to imagine what life would be like for her if we did it. We didn't know if she'd ever get out of the hospital if we didn't. My friends tried to comfort and reassure me. They said she'd always be the same vivacious, compassionate, and kind person—that she'd be the same Dalia—even if she couldn't speak. They assured me she'd find new ways to communicate, that she wouldn't lose her voice even if she could no longer talk.

Kind and thoughtful sentiments, but not convincing. We weren't ready to give in, to admit that we couldn't heal our daughter. We wanted almost more than anything to give her some relief, to see her stop struggling and go home. *Almost* more than anything. What we really wanted was to rewind and go back to our lives pre-hospital, pre-Florida, pre-pneumonia. We were still kidding ourselves that might happen.

We convened a meeting of everyone involved in her care. We wanted to get all the specialists in one room to hash it out and see if we could come to a consensus. We were amazed so many people showed up. Seated around the table were Dr. Navinsky, Pat O'Malley, the pulmonologist, the speech therapist, the mitochondrial specialist, and three of the lead nurses—two of whom came in on their day off to join the meeting.

Rob and I believed if we had even one person on our side, one expert who felt there was a chance Dalia could get better without the surgery, it was worth waiting. The conversation went around and around. This one said we could wait as long as we wanted, but it was a foregone conclusion she'd end up with the trach. He'd seen it play out that way too many times. That one said it was too big a gamble to wait, that we were risking a crisis she wouldn't be able to recover from.

Finally, Dr. Navinsky had his say. I braced myself for more details on the nightmare of life with a trach he'd mentioned earlier. "In general, I'm a pessimist," he began. "So I think most people in this room will be surprised to hear that I think Dalia deserves more time. The first time I saw this little girl I saw a light in her eyes. And I've seen it every day since. She's telling the world that she has a spark and the energy to give this fight everything she has."

Who was going to argue with that? The team agreed to give her one more week to see if she could regain enough strength to start swallowing, clearing her lungs, and breathing independently for a sustained period.

We began a new kind of vigil. To the casual visitor, it would seem the days revolved around therapies and art projects and the movie *Rio*, which Dalia insisted on watching at least three times a day for the fifty-six days we'd been in the hospital. But really what we were doing was holding our breath.

We asked our Jewish friends and our Christian friends and our Muslim friends to pray for her. We even considered making some Buddhist friends so we would have every religion covered. We coddled her even more than we did before. One of us massaged her feet while the other rubbed her forehead. The boys came to visit, crawled into bed with her, and made her laugh. Theo took Dalia's hand and helped her swat him, since she was too weak to do it by herself. She thought that was hysterical. He made himself tumble out of her bed and fall on the floor.

But none of it mattered. Because each day Dalia became a bit weaker. She needed constant suctioning and treatments to move the junk in her lungs.

Four days after the group meeting, Dalia's lung collapsed.

We remembered how the doctor said weeks before that if we listened closely, Dalia would tell us what she needed. Dalia's symptoms would give us our answer. And though we wanted to cover our ears and drown out what we were hearing, we knew Dalia was telling us it was time for a tracheostomy. Her lungs were no longer able to do what they needed to keep her alive.

I didn't want to give in. Giving in felt like we were giving up on the idea that she could recover. I'd prided myself on being able to make things happen. We'd gotten the babies we'd dreamt of. We'd gotten that medical flight back from Florida. We were on our way to getting admitted to the drug trial. But I couldn't make this one thing happen. I couldn't make Dalia's lungs stronger.

Years later, I was on a walk with my neighbor Cheryl—a powerhouse mother, owner of an international PR agency, and yoga instructor—talking about the session she'd taught that morning. "It was a great class," she said. "We talked about the idea of surrender and how surrendering is the opposite of defeat. There's great strength in knowing when to surrender to the flow of life and let it unfold naturally."

By then I understood what she meant. The hardest decision Rob and I ever made—and possibly the one that required the most strength—was to agree to the tracheostomy. But huddled with Rob then, admitting that it was time for a trach felt like massive defeat.

We were each hesitant to bring it up, afraid to be first to capitulate to something we knew we needed to do.

We lay quietly, listening to Dalia's labored breathing.

"We need to do this, right?" I asked Rob.

"I think so," he said.

That was it. We were well past pros and cons and consults and second and third opinions. Rob got up, went over to Dalia's bed, and squeezed in next to her. I went to go find the doctor and tell her what we'd decided.

The operation was scheduled for the following day. As soon as it was over, even before the anesthesia had worn off, we could see Dalia was more comfortable. When she woke up, she wasn't upset. Yes, she was still heavily medicated, but her body was finally, after all these months, able to relax a bit.

All was surprisingly calm until a resident came to clean out Dalia's ears, which had been bothering her for a few days. Somehow, doing something so basic he could have simply used a cotton swab, he lacerated Dalia's ear. Dalia became obsessed with that wound and was nearly oblivious to the trach. Now we had an ailment we could all easily understand. A cut in the ear! This was something we knew how to deal with. We railed and roared and banned that resident from having anything to do with Dalia's care in the future. Here, finally, was a villain we could see. We applied gentle pressure and carefully wiped the wound with antibiotic cream.

Months of deliberation leading to a devastating, life-changing operation, and the thing we all focused on was a cut in Dalia's ear. Maybe it was just the distraction Dalia needed, and for that I'm grateful to the resident. Maybe it was that the ear cut was an injury she could absorb, while the trach was too big a change to contemplate. She wasn't the only one who couldn't fully comprehend it. It was too big for us too.

19

Dressed to Impress

Three days after the tracheostomy, we found out Dalia's cells responded positively to EPI-743, and we were accepted into the research study. Except. Now Dalia was in the hospital, and everything was uncertain. We didn't know what was going to happen in her little body hour to hour, let alone whether she'd be stable enough to participate in a drug trial.

I had to tell NIH what was happening with Dalia, but I was terrified we'd lose our coveted spot in the study. I tried to minimize it, to focus on how well Dalia was doing post-surgery. But the exclamation-point level of enthusiasm from our initial communications dulled immediately. Now the emails from NIH had words like "hopeful," "realistic," "stable enough to travel." They told us to be in touch when Dalia was back home and got her strength back.

We'd convinced ourselves that this drug was the panacea we'd been waiting for. We completely disregarded the fact that the drug was experimental and that even as a participant in the study Dalia had only a fifty-fifty chance of actually getting the drug from the outset, since half of the patients would be getting a placebo. Instead, we allowed ourselves to dream that with this drug Dalia would walk—or even run—again and live a full, healthy life.

I thought of flying out to Stanford to meet with the drug manufacturers to plead our case. I briefly considered what it would take to break into the lab and steal the drug. I wondered if I was too old and tired to successfully proposition one of the researchers.

Rob and I were invited to a MitoAction fundraiser that two of the key doctors working on the drug would be attending. By this point, we'd been in the hospital for almost three months, and I'd embraced a daily uniform of yoga pants and a T-shirt. But I pulled out all the stops for the fundraiser, getting a blowout and manicure and digging a designer dress out of the back of my closet. I changed in the hospital room and headed out.

The whole drive to the party Rob and I planned what we would say to the doctors.

"I want to make sure they know how sweet and brave she is," Rob said.

"Agreed, but let's make sure they understand how healthy she's been up until now. I made a little photo album so they can get a visual."

"You are not going to pull out a photo album at this cocktail party," Rob said.

"Are you kidding? Of course I am. I've got a video, too, if they're up for it."

We arrived at the party and surreptitiously started trying to figure out who the doctors were. We made polite conversation with a few people, while looking over their shoulders to find people who looked doctorly. We were operating on months of sleep deprivation, so it took us longer than it probably should have to realize we could just ask the hostess.

I worried the doctors wouldn't want to engage in serious conversation like this at a cocktail party—that they'd be suspect of this weepy mom waving photos of her daughter trying to assert herself in between the passed hors d'oeuvres and witty repartee they'd been enjoying. But they weren't only polite, they were actually interested in our story. They wanted to hear about Dalia and how her cells had responded to their drug in the lab. Their goal was to bring their drug to market. They needed patients like Dalia to help them make their case.

"I don't see any reason a trach should get in the way of her participating," the first doctor said.

"I agree," said the second. "But ultimately we don't choose the participants; that's up to NIH."

I felt like we'd been victorious, that a personal connection would surely benefit us. Our work was done, so we grabbed a couple of mushroom puffs and headed back to the hospital. Rob dropped me at the front lobby and headed home to relieve the babysitter.

My heels tapped a metronome across the linoleum when I walked into the PICU entrance.

"Excuse me, ma'am. Can I see your ID?" Teresa at the front desk asked.

"Um, sure. Teresa, it's me—Jessie." I slowed to face her, gesturing a circle around my face.

"Oh my word. Jessie! You clean up nice, my friend," she said, chuckling. "You're all set, go on in."

The next day I wrote to NIH letting them know about my conversation with the doctors. I shared how enthusiastic they'd been and reiterated that we'd be leaving the hospital soon and would surely be up for driving the seven and a half hours it would take us to get to NIH if Dalia's new health status prevented her from flying. They said Dalia's name was still on the list and that we'd most likely join the next cycle of patients, which would start in a few months.

I needed more reassurance. "Does that mean we're in?" I emailed. The response from the lead doctor at NIH was immediate.

> My optimistic heart wants to say, "Yes for sure," but my realistic doctor side says, "It means as long as she stays stable to travel and I still have spots to fill, she's in." The only scenario I can imagine is if she were to have another issue and not be able to travel for the trial. I can't "hold" a spot for her, but I have no problem with her even being in the last group to start, which we expect to likely be in fall. So, let's see how she does once she is at home and see how she heals over the next bit of time. I think this is still really good news.

Part of me knew I should prepare for the worst, assume she wouldn't be able to participate, and be pleasantly surprised if she was admitted. But that approach went against the very core of my being. I believed in hope intertwined with action.

At every Passover seder my father read from a piece he wrote: "How do we keep hope alive? The tradition teaches that we are *asirei tikvah*—prisoners of hope. Hope is a curious prison, a prison without walls. In the words of Dr. Martin Luther King Jr., 'We must accept finite disappointment, but never lose infinite hope.' That is what it means to be a prisoner of hope."

But hope didn't feel like a prison to me. The absence of hope seemed far more punishing. And yet, hope on its own felt too passive. I believed if I could make our story compelling enough, beg powerfully enough, they'd agree. I wasn't willing or able to sit back and let hope and luck steer the way.

20

The Stuff

The day before Dalia left the hospital, I was home alone, planning to get Dalia's room in order–to make sure it still felt homey and not like a hospital room.

I paced up and down our driveway waiting for the deliveries, which were arranged by the hospital, when three trucks pulled into our driveway. *This seems a bit excessive. Is it possible the hospital sent food and flowers too?*

Two guys jumped out of the first truck and unloaded a hospital bed. It was so junky, like the cots we slept in at camp, but with side rails. Made of metal, with a fake scratched wood veneer on each end, it had a cracker-thin mattress and a huge hand crank to raise and lower the frame.

The next person emerged from his truck with what looked like a medieval torture device or a prop from *Fifty Shades of Grey*. About four and a half feet tall and six feet long, it was made of thick black metal and had big chains hanging from it. It weighed more than one hundred pounds, and the muscly delivery guy struggled to get it up the stairs and into the bedroom. When I asked what it was, he told me it was a Hoyer lift, meant to lift a person... in the same vein as, say, a crane. I asked him to remove it. It took up nearly all the floor space in the room and didn't exactly go with the pink and purple butterfly décor. For now at least, we'd be just fine to lift our daughter with our arms.

He returned to the truck and came out with four oxygen tanks of various sizes. He carried them in gingerly and warned me to put them somewhere easily accessible yet totally removed from any activity that could knock them over, lest they explode. I was just trying to figure that one out—at hand's length but also out of reach—when another guy walked in with a hand truck loaded with boxes. I counted as he stacked them in Dalia's room; there were five. He went back and forth, loading and unloading more boxes, for a total of thirty-three. The last person carried in a food pump, two ventilators, and an oximeter. I signed the paperwork, and the trucks drove away.

I went back to Dalia's room, plopped down in the middle of thirty-three boxes of I had no idea what, looked at the hideous bed, and silently wept.

But there was little time for that. I needed to make some semblance of order out of the boxes of stuff so the room would feel good to Dalia when she got home.

Six of those boxes contained gauze. There was gauze that measured four inches by four inches and gauze that measured two by two. There was "split gauze," "drainage gauze," and "dressing gauze," "woven gauze" and "non-woven gauze." There was gauze that was meant to be placed around Dalia's new feeding tube and gauze that would tuck under the trach.

There were three boxes of syringes of mixed sizes and three of various-sized suction catheters. There was more stuff in Dalia's room now than in an entire Guatemalan *farmacia*.

There was tubing in a variety of diameters and lengths. Each of the two ventilators had unique tubing attachments.

There was soft-ended tubing and hard-ended tubing, tubes to get stuff into the body and tubes to take other stuff out. The indecipherable diagrams on the paper inserts brought me right back to my post-college Ikea furniture days. Warnings that the tubing needed to be changed every two weeks were printed on the packaging.

There were nearly one hundred cans of PediaSure and boxes filled with two different kinds of bags to use with the food pump. There were boxes of water. Bottles of sterile water and bags of water, which I would later learn were for adding moisture to the ventilator. There were HMEs (heat moisture exchangers) for the trach, which I recognized from the hospital, and HMEs for the vent, which I could only identify as plastic thingamajigs. There were spare trachs and spare G-tubes, mouth sponges and saline bullets.

There was a nebulizer to administer certain medications directly into the lungs and a cough assist device, which is a machine with a long tube (more tubing!) that's placed over the trach to push air in and suck air out to help move secretions out of the lungs. There was a mister, which sits over the trach and provides moisture. It came with fifty feet of its own tubing.

I didn't know what most of the stuff was. I couldn't—and didn't want to—imagine that Dalia needed it and that I'd have to learn how to use it all. The tubing alone was so intimidating, I wanted to marry Rob all over again when he told me he would be the tubing guy and I would never have to deal with any of it.

Did that make me a coward? How could I let tubing scare me when Dalia was dealing with the fact that she could no longer speak or eat? I wanted to breathe in her bravery, to face my relatively small challenges in as dignified a manner as she was facing her huge ones.

But I didn't know if I could. I was scared—scared I'd never know the difference between split gauze and dressing gauze, scared I'd knock over an oxygen tank, scared I'd mix up the tubing, scared that my daughter needed all this equipment, scared that I wasn't up to the task of caring for her.

But I didn't have time to wallow. I didn't have time to let the fear paralyze me.

Because there was one thing I was confident about. I knew I could organize the hell out of that room and make it the best non-hospital-looking, medically tricked-out bedroom ever. That was a challenge I was ready to embrace head-on, so I got out my label maker and got to work.

PART THREE

Ready or Not

21

Homecoming

Dalia was discharged from the hospital on a gorgeous day in May, the polar opposite of the snowy evening when she was admitted several months earlier. As we wheeled Dalia out of the PICU, doctors and nurses lined both sides of the hallways and cheered. "Bye, Dalia!" "Good luck!" "We love you!" Dalia mouthed, "My going home," over and over in response. I hugged the nurses and said, "Don't take this personally, but we hope we never see you again."

Our minivan was packed with dozens of bags of ephemera accumulated during our three-month-stay. Clothes, stuffed animals, books, and art projects filled one-half of the back. A ventilator, oxygen tanks, and a brand-new wheelchair filled the other.

I rode next to Dalia, steadying her in a booster seat. She'd lost so much muscle tone during her three months in bed that she needed to be propped up or she'd flop right over. Rob drove dangerously below the speed limit on the Mass Pike, while I monitored Dalia's trach and oxygenation and heart rate. The windows were open. Loose strands of Dalia's hair broke free of her braids and blew in the breeze.

I wasn't used to this version of Dalia—quiet, serene. Before, Dalia's silliness and mischief took up the entire back seat. She'd put her hand over her window when she caught Theo looking out. "My window," she giggled, blocking his view. She'd ask Rob to go "super rocket," pushing a pretend accelerator to tell him to speed up. When we passed the farm near our house she'd roll down her window and yell, "Thank you, cows, for the ice cream!"

Now she gazed outside, looking so much more relaxed than I felt.

There was a piece of me that felt like we were bringing home a new baby. We were overwhelmed and sleep deprived and surprised anybody thought we were responsible enough to care for such a dependent person, exactly how my friends told me they felt when they left the hospital with their newborns.

The difference was that with a new baby, friends and family can help, cheer you on, and even babysit.

We were flying solo here. There wasn't one person in our lives who could remotely relate to what we were going through. There was nobody to give us useful advice or meaningful reassurance or even to take a turn at suctioning Dalia's secretions—something that needed to be done several times an hour. Once again, we had to be the experts. The only problem was we had no idea what we were doing.

We had fifteen medications to keep track of that had to be dosed into syringes and given at different times throughout the day. We had to figure out what all the machines were, which alarms were actually alarming and which were merely annoying, and how to safely move Dalia around the house with all the tubes and machines that were attached to her. We had to give her all her food and water and meds via her new feeding tube and learn when to suction her trach, her nose, and her mouth.

When we left the hospital, we were told that after an extended stay like ours nearly half of all patients return within forty-eight hours.

But it was the first time the five of us were together in the house in months, and we were determined to inject a bit of normalcy. The boys had borne the brunt of our exhaustion and anxiety and absence. Their lives were spinning out of control, too, and we were desperate to tell them—and show them—that the nightmare was over.

That first Sunday at home was Mother's Day. My favorite way to spend Mother's Day is to have breakfast with the kids and spend the day by myself. I want no motherly responsibilities, which is a bit ironic given how many Mother's Days I spent longing to be able to bask in maternal glory.

But this year was different. Neither Rob nor I was comfortable being with Dalia without the other in earshot. And the very idea that being alone with our nine-year-old was a terrifying proposition was all the proof we needed that the "normal" we'd returned to was an entirely new one.

We invited our family for a cookout. To a certain extent, it was a regular family get-together. The boys pushed Dalia in her wheelchair, chasing their five-year-old cousin Marisol with water guns. My father fell asleep in the middle of dinner. Theo ate four turkey dogs and two pieces of chicken. A bird pooped in my hair. Perfectly normal.

But beneath the veneer of this Rockwellian holiday was a slightly off-kilter Picasso effect.

When my niece Marisol arrived with her parents, she ran up to the deck as always. Dalia saw Marisol coming and started kicking her legs in excitement, mouthing, "Marisol here, Marisol here." But as soon as Marisol saw Dalia, she stopped short. She grasped her mother's hand and looked at Dalia with her mouth slightly open, noticing the strange-looking tube coming out of Dalia's neck, snaking down the front of her body and attached to a hissing machine. Her mother, Aliette, gently prodded her, "It's okay *guapa*. You can give Dalia a hug." And sweet Marisol approached Dalia to gingerly embrace her. There it was: The first indication that people would see Dalia differently. Our new sad normal.

After a couple hours of playing, we set out our Mother's Day feast. I planned a casual barbecue rather than a sit-down meal, on the theory that a seated dinner would exclude Dalia, who couldn't eat anymore. Her meals were all the same, a single can of PediaSure that went through her G-tube directly to her stomach, bypassing her taste buds altogether.

But whether we were milling about barbecue-style or at a seated table was irrelevant to Dalia. I set out a huge bowl of potato chips, forgetting that potato chips were Dalia's favorite. As soon as she saw the chips, she started pointing at them. She couldn't talk anymore but she could point with more vehemence than a shout, and she was pointing loudly—screamingly—at those chips. I watched as it dawned on her that it wasn't just that she *hadn't* eaten in months; it was that she *couldn't* eat anymore.

"I want some, I want some," Dalia mouthed. We all descended, rushing in to try to distract her. Theo handed her a water gun, while Jonah quickly moved the chips. Rob brought out the singing balloon a neighbor dropped off a few hours before. My dad told a joke, "It happened in Minsk, or maybe it was Pinsk," he began. I wiped the tears streaming down my face and started reading *Don't Let the Pigeon Drive the Bus* aloud in a quivering voice. We were rookies—each of us doing our best, all of us at a loss.

22

It's My Party and I'll Cry

Dalia turned nine in the hospital. We did what we could to make it festive: balloons, presents, music. But no amount of feigned festivity could mask the fear and exhaustion we felt. So we promised her the biggest, best birthday party she could imagine when she got home.

We had seventy-eight days in the hospital to imagine the party before she was released from the PICU, and each week the vision became more elaborate. Nurse Karen suggested we get a petting zoo. Nurse Liz said we should get a band, and Nurse Melissa voted for carnival rides.

We were up for all of it. There were so many days when we questioned whether she'd leave the hospital at all, days when we didn't see any progress or even worse, days when things seemed to be moving backward. Those were the times when one of the nurses or a visiting friend would try to cheer us up. "Let's talk about the party," they'd say, and they'd do their best to get our minds out of the hospital and into a gorgeous summer day when all our family and friends would be together celebrating Dalia.

As soon as we got home, I began putting the plans in motion. In so many ways I didn't know how to take care of Dalia. But I knew how to throw a party, and I wasn't going to sacrifice any amount of indulgence or excess. Birthday parties are a celebration of life, and if any life deserved celebrating it was Dalia's.

The party was still six weeks away, so I found the *Farmer's Almanac* online to make sure the day I picked was predicted to be sunny. I knew how crazy that was, but in a world where everything was spinning out of control, I thought maybe I could at least try to control the weather.

I pored over menus and weighed cooking versus catering and finally decided to go with a sushi-fest. "Why don't we just order pizza instead and be done with it?" Rob asked. I added pizza to the menu, because who doesn't enjoy a slice with their California roll? Rob started brewing beers, and I researched frozen cocktails we could make in a Vitamix. Then I bought a Vitamix.

Dalia, of course, wouldn't be able to partake in any of the food or beverages, but I wanted the menu to be fabulous, nonetheless. The party was more than just a celebration of Dalia—it was also a thank-you to everyone who had been by our side for the three months we were in the hospital.

I hired a face painter and a balloonist, things I knew Dalia would enjoy. Then I decided I needed something for the adults, too, so I added a caricature artist and lawn games to the mix.

I began making daily trips to Target to buy all the essentials and tons of things that were nonessential but looked good. I decided an ice cream sundae bar would be fun, but the day before the party I realized it was going to be ninety degrees and no amount of ice would keep the ice cream in a solid state, so I called five ice cream stores until I found one that would lend me a chest freezer.

I spent seven hours crafting the perfect playlist, passing each song through the "Jonah test" to make sure it was cool. I decluttered and scrubbed and organized the house. I bought a dress and got a blowout and a mani-pedi.

And then, when the day of the party finally arrived, I woke up at 6:00 a.m. to start the real preparation.

By 2:00, everything was set up perfectly. "Come check it out, sweetie," I said, wheeling Dalia from the welcome signs to the balloonist to croquet. She smiled and pointed from one thing to the next, taking in the way our front yard was transformed into a summer wonderland. An hour left before the guests were to arrive, we had Dalia's portrait drawn and watched the balloonist make her a small zoo's worth of latex animals. Then, at 2:45, Dalia's eyelids began to close.

I'd taken almost every contingency into consideration. But somehow, the one thing I neglected to think about was that Dalia was recovering from several major surgeries and the trauma of months in a hospital bed. Not to mention the fact that her underlying condition itself, MERRF syndrome, was an energy deficiency disease. Going to see *Frozen* at the movie theater exhausted her.

The guests started to arrive: Rachel and my dad and the rest of the family, colleagues, our friends, and the kids' friends. A couple of nurses from the PICU even showed up.

The yard was overflowing with essentially everyone we'd ever known, and each person wanted to see Dalia. I could tell from their faces how much they knew before they'd arrived. There were the quivery smiles of the people who weren't prepared for the changes. They looked away and hoped we didn't catch the tears in their eyes. Then there were the huge grins of those who had been by our side at the hospital. They didn't hide their tears of joy.

The heat was oppressive, especially for Dalia, who had trouble regulating her body temperature. We could tell by looking at the numbers on the ventilator that the volume of air she was taking into her lungs was lower than it was supposed to be. But we didn't need to see the machine display to know that. In the hospital, the nurses taught us to "look at the patient, not the numbers." One look at Dalia and we knew she wasn't doing well. Her face was red, her eyes nearly closed, and her head was leaning to the side, like the extended neck stretch we did in my yoga class.

"Should we put her in bed?" I asked Rob. "Let me see if I can cool her off under a tree," he suggested, neither of us wanting to remove the guest of honor from her own party. Rob and Dalia spent most of the day on the sidelines, Rob holding a cold compress on Dalia's forehead, measuring her oxygen, and taking her temperature every few minutes.

We'd been looking forward to the party for months, but clearly, I overdid it. In my rush to compensate for everything Dalia went through, I threw the party I wanted, not the one that made sense for her. It was healthy for all of us to have something fun to look forward to, and I also wanted to create great memories to look back on. I wanted to stuff so many good memories in the coffer that they'd squeeze out the bad ones.

More and more I felt like Fred Flintstone with the angel and devil on my shoulders, only in my case the angel was my inner optimist and the devil was the pessimist. Optimist said we'd find a cure, we'd beat the odds, we'd throw the best birthday party in the history of parties. Pessimist crossed her arms in front of her chest, lifted an eyebrow, and asked, "Who are you kidding?"

— ⸎ —

Later that night, after all the guests left and the overnight nurse arrived, Rob and I lay in bed debriefing.

What he said: "Great party. I think everyone had a really good time. I just wish Dalia hadn't been so tired."

What he meant: "Why the hell was Dalia so tired? She was barely awake during the entire thing."

What I said: "Yeah, I think it went well. Do you think she had a good time?"

What I meant: "I couldn't tell if she enjoyed it at all. I wish she hadn't seemed so out of it."

What he said: "Of course. How could she not have had a good time? Nobody throws a party like you do."

What neither of us said: "This is so fucking scary."

Neither one of us wanted to introduce our fears right then, to risk bringing the other one down if we weren't in the same headspace. And besides, saying our fears out loud might transform them from our own individual dark imaginings to real possibilities.

"I'm going to get some water," Rob said, getting out of bed. A few seconds later I heard a thud from the hallway outside our room. "Sorry. Dropped a book," Rob called back to me.

But he hadn't dropped a book. In the morning he went to the emergency room to have his hand x-rayed. He'd broken it punching a doorframe. What was disarming wasn't that Rob was terrified. We'd lived so long with our fear it had become like an annoying roommate. Some nights it kept us up, some mornings it woke us early. What was unnerving was that his fear looked so wildly different from mine. I overcompensated, pushed the fear to the fringes. Rob pushed his down, and then it came flooding out as anger.

23

House of Mirrors

On top of everything else, there was now a troupe of strangers in and out of our house every day.

Dalia was an "eyes-on" patient, meaning Rob or I or a nurse trained specifically in Dalia's care needed to have our eyes on her every minute of the day and night. The good news was we were given one hundred hours of nursing per week paid for by the state of Massachusetts. There is no conceivable way we would have been able to afford the nursing hours—or the medications and medical supplies for that matter—without the state's support.

The bad news was we were at the mercy of a nursing agency to find people to fill all those hours and there was a national nursing shortage.

The nursing agency sent people to check on the nurses, and the company that supplied the medical equipment stopped by to make sure it was working. There were also personal care attendants to supplement the nursing hours.

I made a color-coded spreadsheet to remember who was meant to be in the house when, but we'd still bump into strangers on the way into the kitchen or coming out of the bathroom. I couldn't walk around the house without wearing a bra anymore. I had to strike "motherfucker" from my vocabulary at precisely the time when it felt most useful.

But I was grateful for the strangers, some of whom began to feel like family. We were in so far over our heads that I would have welcomed my mechanic to come stay a while if he could change ventilator tubing. Forget going braless, I'd have worn a corset if it meant an extra set of hands that knew what they were doing.

The problem was our team was a mixed bag.

Erin was an experienced nurse. She was with us only on Tuesdays, which soon became our favorite night because we knew we'd sleep soundly, confident that Dalia was in excellent hands. Until the night she called us from Dalia's room at 2:00 a.m.

"I think there's a burglar in the house," she whispered. "I hear someone creeping around."

Rob ran to the garage to get a baseball bat. I ran to Theo's and Jonah's rooms to see which of them had been playing a trick on Erin.

"I'm sure it wasn't the boys," Erin said when I told her my theory. "Listen, I recorded it," she said, hitting "play" on her phone. "Hellooooo . . . Hellooooo . . . Hellooooo."

"Erin, I'm thinking a burglar probably wouldn't say 'hello,'" I said.

She considered that and tentatively agreed. "Okay, but the only way I'm comfortable staying here is if you leave the baseball bat with me just in case."

The next day our rep from the nursing agency called. "I don't know how to tell you this; it's a new one for us. Erin thinks there's paranormal activity in your home, so she won't be returning."

We had another nurse who told us after her first shift with Dalia that she believed Rob and I were God's soldiers and that our house was holy ground. She alternated between looking through Dalia's paperwork and reading the Bible, forgoing any task that had to do with actual nursing. I guess she assumed God was taking care of that part of her job.

My favorite might have been the nurse who told us there was a stomach bug going around, and if Dalia or any member of our family was showing symptoms, she wasn't coming to work. She was a nurse. The very purpose of her job was to take care of sick people. That would be like a police officer refusing to work in a high-crime area.

Dalia was back in school now, accompanied each day by a private nurse. We hired Viola for the job. She taught in a school in Kenya before she emigrated to the United States, and her dream was to return there to open a school of her own. She was a strong woman who could lift Dalia's sixty-five pounds effortlessly, and I was prepared to love her. The only thing stopping me was that she was sleeping on the job.

One day the school nurse called me. "We're concerned about Viola," she said. "She's fallen asleep a few times while Dalia's doing classwork."

Obviously this wasn't ideal, but we were beholden to her. I have friends who ignore the fact that their kids' babysitters spend the whole night on the phone or always show up late, because it would be so hard to replace them. This was that, only the stakes were much higher. Without Viola, Dalia wouldn't be able to go to school, which would be yet another loss for her. It would also mean I wouldn't be able to work, and I'd only just returned. "Let's give her another chance," I said. "Maybe she's just resting with her eyes closed."

But a few days later, Jonah returned from school to find Viola sleeping in our living room—while Dalia was in her bedroom on a different floor of the house. Viola was done.

She wasn't the only nurse to sleep on the job, though. Sleeping was endemic to the night nurses. There was Morgan, who we found not only sleeping, but with headphones in. Rob had to nudge her toe twice to wake her up so he could fire her. She showed up the next night for her shift, as though she'd dreamt what happened the night before.

We replaced Morgan with Inga, but on her third night Rob found her sound asleep, curled up under a blanket, and snoring.

I was already asleep when Rob came into our bedroom to grab his pillow.

"Inga was asleep. I'll see you in the morning."

I followed him into Dalia's room, where he was settling in for the night on the chair by her bed.

"I think maybe we should consider giving the nurses a second chance when they fall asleep. I don't think we can afford to keep losing them," I said, without looking at Rob.

"That's bullshit," he said, looking right at me. "Their only job is to be awake."

"Right, but it's not good for you to stay up and then go to work tomorrow. Can we at least give them one strike before they're out?"

"What . . . and risk our daughter's life?"

I went back to bed and lay awake. I wasn't sure why it bothered me so much that Rob fired the nurse, since he was also the one who would lose sleep over it. I felt selfish for wanting to sleep, and I thought Rob was being sanctimonious. There was no way for me to respond when he pulled the "risk our daughter's life" card.

— ◊◊ —

I felt judged, and I felt it from everyone who had a front-row seat to the inner workings of our family. People were there when we were feeling vulnerable and just wanted to curl up and cry. They were there when we were frustrated and wanted to scream and swear and punch the wall.

I wondered if they were judging me when I served cereal for dinner or told our boys it was fine to skip showering . . . for the third night in a row. I wondered what they thought about Rob's favorite way to get the boys out of bed in the morning—blasting Ozzy Osbourne's "Crazy Train" from the speakers in their rooms. I feared that a nurse returned home at night and said to her sister, "You wouldn't believe what a mess that house is. Every surface in the living room is covered in unfolded laundry." Which was true, but none of their business.

Once a nurse actually did make her judgment crystal clear though, and it was on a topic I didn't see coming. Her email was addressed solely to me:

> Dalia's needs require your full attention. In my thirty years of nursing, I've never seen a child with needs as complex as Dalia's where a family member isn't present at all times. When you're with Dalia, if you're thinking about work, you are risking Dalia's safety. I tell you this because I think if you keep going this way, it's only a matter of time before something catastrophic happens. I myself chose decades ago to give up a big career to stay home and care for my children, and I never regretted it for a second. I understand if you choose to ignore this advice, but I wouldn't be able to live with myself if I didn't tell you how I felt.

She didn't offer similar advice to Rob, even though I was the primary breadwinner and Rob was a better caregiver. I read the email to Rob.

"It sounds like she's struggling with her own decision. Anyway, why do you care what she thinks?" he said.

I forwarded the email to Rachel. "That's crazy, Jess; she's completely out of line. You need to fire her."

But what if she was right? Would Dalia have a better chance at recovery if I quit my job? I didn't see how my being home would make a difference, particularly since Dalia was at school all day. *But maybe I should be there when she got home from school?* Maybe I was more stressed or distracted because of my job and wasn't giving Dalia the attention her condition demanded.

I didn't consider taking Rachel's advice to fire the nurse. Instead, I thanked the nurse for sharing her thoughts and told her I'd see her the next morning before I left for work. The energy it would take to engage on this and the risk of losing a highly qualified and committed nurse weren't worth it. But I wasn't able to shake it off, not because it was inappropriate and ballsy, which it was, but because it reinforced the nascent fear that whatever I gave to my kids—and Dalia in particular—could never be enough.

24

Getting Schooled

Most of the nurses didn't think our house had paranormal activity or fall asleep on the job. The majority were professional. But every once in a while someone would show up at our house with so much calmness or competence or creativity they made everyone else seem dull by comparison.

Shawna was twenty-three. She looked like a Kardashian and had a cool, tough veneer like Angelina Jolie mixed with wrestler Ronda Rousey. Her arms were covered in tattoos, her nose pierced, and her fingernails so long I could hear them clicking on her phone from the next room. She did not exude Mary Poppins-ness.

If you had told me the day we met her that Shawna would become Dalia's best friend, I'd have laughed out loud.

Dalia's first real playdate, years before, had been with a friend named Karla. Dalia was already using a walker, and we struggled getting up the stairs that led to Karla's front door. As Dalia and I walked into the house, Karla's mother moved two small chairs out of the way and then ran upstairs to grab a basket of toys so Dalia wouldn't need to climb to the second-level playroom. The next time we decided to get the girls together at our house. Karla ran from room to room doing a quick pass to see what toys we had. Then she did a second, slower loop before settling in our third-floor loft. But after five minutes there, she wanted to go play in Dalia's room, then downstairs to check out the treats, then back up to the loft. Dalia simply couldn't keep up. That was the last playdate we had with Karla. It was deflating for Dalia and exhausting for me.

And that was before the wheelchair.

Most homes aren't wheelchair accessible. Ours wasn't until two years after Dalia was in a chair. At first, we invited Dalia's classmates to our house, where Dalia would be more comfortable. But as Dalia became weaker, her friends became stronger. They were running and doing cartwheels and playing hide-and-go-seek. Dalia was losing her ability to walk.

The last birthday party I took Dalia to was at Jump Nation, whose name alone suggests how inappropriate it was for Dalia. I knew it was a gamble, but Dalia begged to go. As soon as we arrived, Dalia fixated on the inflated slide that took up a third of the room. To reach the top of the slide, you had to climb up a set of bouncy stairs—kind of challenging even for someone with two legs that worked perfectly.

I stood behind Dalia, my arms under hers, and clumsily carried her up those stairs time and time again so she could sit on my lap and ride down the slide with the other kids. The other moms sat on benches that lined the walls, chatting or scrolling on their phones. I hated that party. I envied the moms their time off, and I resented all the able-bodied kids who whined about the long lines.

Even the quiet activities became more difficult for Dalia. Her tremoring hands hampered her ability to hold a game piece or a paintbrush. After she got the trach tube, the playdates stopped altogether.

– ≫ ≪ –

Dalia missed three months of school when she was in the hospital, and she'd miss another few recovering, so the school district sent a teacher from school to tutor her a few times a week. The first time Shawna walked through our door, Dalia recognized her and hung her head in dismay. I'm not sure if it was Shawna in particular or Dalia's realization that she didn't get a six-month no-homework pass, but either way she was not a gracious hostess.

Shawna pulled a small whiteboard and magnetic letters out of her backpack.

"Dalia, can you point to the letters in your name?"

Dalia crossed her arms and looked away.

"Nice try, Dalia. I know you know how to spell your name."

Dalia closed her eyes.

"Maybe we need to change her hearing aid batteries," I said.

"She woke up early today," Rob said. "I think she needs a rest."

"Well, it's too bad that Dalia's so sleepy," Shawna said. "Because now I'll have to give these unicorn stickers to Theo."

Dalia's eyes sprang open, and she pointed to the magnetic D. I made a mental note to stock up on unicorn stickers.

Shawna started spending more and more time at our house. When she and Dalia finished their lessons, Shawna played videos on her phone for Dalia—Taylor Swift and Katy Perry and Beyoncé. She choreographed a dance she and Dalia could do using only their shoulders and flipping their hair dramatically. She held Dalia's hand and moved it in sync to the music. The boys thought Shawna was cool. They circled around, asking what she thought of A$AP Rocky or Drake.

One day, the six of us drove to New Hampshire to hang out at Rachel's pool. We brought Dalia's food pump and ventilator and also a bag full of games for Dalia to play with while Jonah and Theo swam.

But Dalia had a different idea. A few minutes after the boys started splashing, Dalia mouthed, "I want to swim."

I looked at Rob. He was looking down. His eyes were red, and I wondered if he was going to cry.

How are we going to tell Dalia it isn't safe for her to go in the pool? That her machines needed to stay dry and her trach tube can't get wet?

I felt like I'd swallowed a concoction of fear and sadness and failure. Why were we punishing our daughter? Imagine taking a young girl to a gorgeous pool on a perfect summer day and making her stay on the sidelines while everybody else jumps in. And there were no alternatives for her. It wasn't like she could ride the merry-go-round while everyone else was on the roller coaster. The games we'd packed were a feeble attempt at distraction.

"I'm cool with it if it's okay with you," Shawna said. "I can hold her on the steps, and she can splash with her feet."

We were quiet for a few seconds while we considered whether this was an audacious offer or an idea we should have come up with ourselves.

"Really? Are you sure?" Rob asked. "Because I can hold the tube and watch the vent if we position it right here," he said, motioning to the edge of the pool stairs.

I wasn't half as strong as Shawna or nearly as confident with the machines as Rob, so my job would be to hold Dalia's hands.

It took ten minutes of coordination, then Shawna positioned herself on the pool stairs and Rob carefully placed Dalia right between Shawna's legs, the water rising to Dalia's belly. Dalia immediately started kicking her legs to splash the boys, who swam right up to her to make sure the splatter reached them.

We came so close to spinning out, but now we were back on track.

Another day, Theo and Dalia were playing Chutes and Ladders.

"Mom, Dalia's cheating," Theo said. "She's supposed to land on the chute, but she's trying to skip over that box."

"Theo, just let her win," I whispered at the exact same time Shawna said, "Dalia, you are such a cheater!" All of us started cracking up. Dalia's silent laugh was the loudest.

Shawna spent hours helping us transform Dalia's wheelchair into a sleigh for Halloween so she could ride in style as Elsa. She plopped into Dalia's bed at naptime and slept beside her, gently moving the feeding tube aside. When Dalia became fixated on getting tattoos like Shawna's, Shawna carefully drew a replica of her tattoos on Dalia's tiny arms. When it was shower time, Dalia demanded that we keep her arms out of the water to preserve Shawna's masterpiece—for two weeks.

I was a sucker when it came to most things Dalia wanted; one Dalia pout and I'd give in. When Jonah finally earned a phone after a year of working toward it, Shawna, Dalia, and I went to the Verizon store to pick it up. As soon as Dalia realized we were there to get a phone for Jonah, she started kicking her legs, clenching her hands into fists, and mouthing, "I want one; I want one." I was ready to give Dalia my old phone. I didn't care that she couldn't talk and her fingers were too shaky to use the keyboard. I couldn't give her stronger muscles or stronger lungs, but I could give her a phone. Shawna looked at me and asked, "Are you crazy?" Then she turned to Dalia. "Dalia," she said, "you'll get a phone when you're thirteen, just like Jonah."

Shawna treated Dalia like a perfectly normal kid, which is probably one of the reasons Dalia adored Shawna so much. Every afternoon when she came home from school, Dalia looked at us and mouthed, "Where's Shawna?"

The adoration went both ways, as evidenced by the huge dahlia flower Shawna had tattooed on her leg with Dalia's handwriting of her own name stenciled underneath. When I asked Shawna what she said when people saw her tattoo and asked her who Dalia is, she replied without hesitation, "My best friend."

I knew why Dalia loved Shawna, but I wasn't sure why Shawna felt so connected to Dalia. One day I asked.

"I love the way she loves," Shawna began. "She's in this horrific situation that she has zero control over, but she worries when Rob gets poison ivy or when the dog is shaking when he goes to the groomer, because she just genuinely loves everybody so much. And when you tell her that we're going to Target or Petco, she starts dancing and acts like it's the most exciting thing that could happen to us. She's the most positive, enthusiastic person I know."

The magic of Shawna rubbed off on each of us. I became braver with Dalia physically, and the boys did too. We stopped treating her like a delicate figurine that was only taken off the shelf for dusting. They saw that it was still okay to get annoyed by her just like they would with a typically developing sister.

Even more important, we learned that we could still be happy, even though we were decimated.

25

Another Best Friend

I have never been a dog person. I didn't grow up with a dog, unless you count Roger, the dog who lived with us for eighteen hours until he pooped on our living room floor and my father brought him back to the store, claiming he was defective and asking for a refund. Rob and I together had raised a golden retriever named Mowgli. I tolerated him, but we never bonded. Once, when we returned from vacation and I went to pick up Mowgli at the Doggie Hotel, they gave us the wrong dog. It took me twenty minutes to realize the mistake.

During our three-month stay in the hospital, a volunteer brought a therapy dog into our room every Thursday to play and snuggle. The dog sat up and put its feet on Dalia's bed, waiting for the treats Dalia loved to dole out. "Nother," Dalia would say, smiling and reaching out her hand to get one more treat. "Nother," she'd say a second time, and then a third.

One time a dog named Stella came to visit, arriving just a few minutes before Dalia was scheduled for an MRI. When the team came to the room to prep Dalia for transport, she wouldn't let go of Stella.

"Okay, darlin'," the nurse said. "Stella can come with us to the exam room if you promise to say goodbye when we get there."

We paraded alongside Dalia and Stella down three floors in the elevator and across two walkways and up another four floors in a second elevator. Everybody we passed waved and cheered Dalia and Stella on. When we got to the MRI room, Dalia held on tight to Stella, wrapping her arms around the dog's belly and clasping her hands together. She refused to let go.

"How about if Stella and I wait right here for you?" Stella's owner said.

"I just couldn't bear to say no to your sweet girl," she said to me when Dalia finally released Stella and was wheeled into the exam room.

It wasn't long before Dalia started campaigning for a dog of her own. It was a short campaign, because at that point Dalia could have lobbied for a unicorn, and we would have figured out how to find her one.

"Of course, sweetie," I promised. "When we get out of the hospital, we'll get a dog."

We wanted to say yes to something, anything, Dalia asked. Rob once accidentally tripped over the med cart and fell on the floor. Dalia asked him to do it again, which he did six times when he saw how it made Dalia crack up.

Most of the time what she was asked was, "When can we go home?" And on that one, we never had an answer that was both acceptable and true.

In the scheme of things, Dalia's request for a dog seemed reasonably small.

That was how we found ourselves headed to Logan Airport to meet my friend Jen, who was flying in from Los Angeles to deliver us a dog.

I'd enlisted Jen for the dog search, who over the next many months sent me videos of dogs she visited in shelters around LA. It felt a bit like online dating, only without the possibility of rejection. When Jen sent me a video of a sweet little poodle mix named Blackie-O, who seemed like a live version of the stuffed doggie Dalia slept with, I shared it with the family.

I showed the video to Jonah and Theo, who fell in love immediately. I showed the video to Rob, who didn't consider him a real dog, since he weighed only fifteen pounds. I showed the video to Dalia, and she looked up at me with her bright brown eyes and said, "My doggie?"

Jen adopted Blackie-O on our behalf, took him home for a few weeks to train him, and booked a cross-country flight for two.

"There they are!" I pointed when we saw Jen coming down the escalator clutching a dog carrier. Dalia, in her wheelchair, gripped Rob's hand on one side and Theo's on the other, kicking her legs in excitement. Her eyes sparkled as she watched Jen's approach, amazed this was actually happening.

The next morning we were on a long walk when Theo realized Blackie-O was slowing down. "Who brought water for him?" Theo asked. Rob and I looked at each other, realizing that despite the ninety-degree temperature, bringing water didn't occur to either of us. Rob picked up Blackie-O, deposited him on Dalia's lap, and proceeded to wheel the two of them back home.

After that, Blackie-O decided he was Dalia's dog. He'd be nice enough to the rest of us, but Dalia was his person.

He started sleeping at the end of Dalia's bed. He walked right next to the wheelchair when he wasn't sitting on her lap, and he barked at any stranger who came too close. When Dalia left the house for the day, Blackie-O watched for her out the window next to the front door until she returned. When the boys came home, Blackie-O barely lifted his head. When Rob and I came through the door, he ignored us altogether. But as soon as he heard Dalia's van pull into the driveway, he leapt up and started thwapping his tail so vigorously I worried it might fly off. When Dalia came through the front door, he stood on his back legs and rested his front ones on the side of her chair. He was so protective of her, as though he knew she needed special protecting. He essentially trained himself to become Dalia's service dog.

We began to take him with us everywhere we went with Dalia and quickly learned that nobody would question the fact that we had a dog with us—even in a "no dogs allowed" setting—if he were sitting on Dalia's lap. Instead, people said how adorable he was. Other kids gathered around and asked if they could pet him. Dalia became the center of attention not because she had a tube coming out of her neck or was in a wheelchair, but because she had the cutest dog in town.

When the other kids ran around outside, Blackie-O sat right by Dalia's side watching. When they played baseball or rode bikes, he sat on Dalia's lap and licked her hand. Everybody else looked for Dalia to fit into their world, but Blackie-O took his place right beside Dalia in hers.

"How does Blackie-O know Dalia needs extra love?" Theo asked me one day. "Dogs just know," I answered. But really, I had no idea. Dalia was the only one in the family who never fed Blackie-O, the only one who couldn't throw the ball for him or rub his belly in the place that made his tail wag. I once read that dogs can read human emotion, so maybe he could tell how full of sweetness she was, even though it was increasingly hard for her to show it. Maybe he stuck by her side not because she needed love, but because she personified it.

26

Suit of Armor

I still wore my armor of to-dos and logistics. Now it was fortified with the strong front I put on for the kids.

But one night after Rob and I were already half asleep, Jonah came into our room.

I could see even in the light of the moon coming through our window that his cheeks were blotchy and his eyes were red.

"What's happening, sweetie? Are you okay?"

He stood at the end of the bed and started breathing faster.

"Something's wrong with me," he said, tears pooling in his eyes. And then he started sobbing.

Oh shit, he's sick. But how sick? Does he have appendicitis or strep throat or his first migraine? Maybe it's blepharitis, which I'd been struggling with for weeks and was as annoying as it sounded.

It took a while for the next words to come, but when they did, they poured.

"I'm so scared about Dalia. I just don't understand why this has to happen to her. She's getting worse, and it makes me so mad. She's the best person I know. Why is this happening? I pray and pray and pray, and she doesn't get better."

And then the kicker.

"But you guys are so strong all the time. I never see you get scared. You seem fine."

My stomach burned. It was clear just how not fine we were.

I stood up and wrapped my arms around Jonah. Now the two of us were bawling, with Rob handing us tissue after tissue, tears streaming down his face too.

"What's the matter with me?" Jonah sobbed.

A few months earlier, I'd gone hiking with some friends. We started up the mountain in a pack, but within twenty minutes I was bringing up the rear. It felt like it was two hundred degrees. I was so proud of myself for remembering to wear a hat, but I hadn't thought to bring water. For a while I could see my friends farther up the path, but I slowed way down as I became nauseous and winded, and then I couldn't see them at all. I sat down on the side of the trail to catch my breath.

How is it possible that I'm the least in shape of this entire group? I thought, as I reached for my cell phone. But there was no reception. *Okay, not only am I the least in shape, but I also definitely can't go another step. Should I go back down to the car? But what if they wait for me at the top? I think I'm going to throw up. Why is nobody else realizing this is the hardest hike in the history of hiking? What's the matter with me?*

"Jessie, are you okay?"

My distress was interrupted by a friend who had doubled back to find me.

"I don't feel well," I said, both relieved and embarrassed.

"Oh, I know. I hike every day, and I'm wiped out too. This is a really tough trail. I threw up after I did it the first time. Let's just sit here until you feel ready, and we'll take it together." I thought she might be humoring me, but I didn't care.

After a few minutes, she reached out her hand to help me up, and we got back on the trail. She had a huge bottle of water, and she gave me sips and poured some over my head. We stopped a few times along the way, sometimes because I was tired and sometimes because she was. Then, an hour or three later, we reached the top.

As I stood there that night with my arms around Jonah, it was clear to me that Rob and I had been working so hard to put on a strong front that we'd left Jonah, and probably Theo, alone on the side of the mountain. We needed to double back and let them know how hard it was for us too.

But to do that, I'd need to take off my armor, and my armor was comfortable. It protected me from the slings and arrows coming at me, so I could take care of everything that needed taking care of. I only loosened it at night when I was done being strong. That's when I'd curl up in the chaise by Dalia's bed and let the sadness in. I was scared to take it off completely, afraid that if I did, I'd dissolve into a puddle and not be able to tend to my kids, my husband, myself.

We hugged Jonah. "Oh honey, I'm so sorry."

"I'm terrified every second of the day," Rob started, his armor clanking to the floor. "I'm scared for all of you, but terrified about what's going on with Dalia because I don't understand it, and I can't do anything to fix it. We've tried not to let you and Theo see how scared we are because we didn't want you to have to be scared. We were trying to take that off you. We're terrified."

"Really?" Jonah asked, crinkling his nose.

"Really," I added.

When Jonah left the room, I turned to Rob.

"We really screwed up."

"Yep . . . maybe it's better that it's out in the open."

He was right. Our kids' childhoods weren't going to be carefree. I wanted to protect them. I wanted to shield them from the pain and the fear and the sadness. I wanted to put on a happy face and sing in the car and do the things other families did. I thought maybe if I did that, they wouldn't notice that nothing in our life was normal.

"The number one rule in our family is that we're always honest with each other," we'd told our kids ever since the first time Jonah swore to us he didn't eat the cupcake while we looked at the chocolate smeared all over his face. Yet here we were, lying to them.

Because the truth is the fear and sadness created hairline fractures in my soul that were getting bigger with time. I didn't want any of the kids, or even Rob, to know I was shattered. I wanted to be whole for all of them. And I didn't realize that being whole meant letting them see where I was broken.

27

Two Worlds

We were living in two worlds. In the first, we were on high alert all the time. What might be run-of-the-mill for other families—a feverish daughter or a bloodshot eye—could send us into a panic involving a team of doctors. We'd seen a cold become a three-month hospital stay, so nothing was too small to freak out about.

In the second world, we were Zen masters. Strep throat or a broken foot? Treatable and temporary. It could be so much worse.

In the first world we knew anything could happen, and we were hypervigilant as we braced for another tragedy. In the second we had a profound understanding that most things that did happen really weren't that bad.

On July 4, those two worlds collided.

Up to that point, we'd been careful not to let Dalia's new medical condition make her feel isolated from the family. We still all went to the movies, but we didn't order popcorn, since she couldn't have any. We made sure that at least one of us sat with her in another room during dinner, since she couldn't eat. We hadn't gone on vacation, because she couldn't fly and because we were scarred from the last trip.

I knew we needed to start thinking about what we were taking away from Jonah and Theo while we were working so hard to protect Dalia.

On July 3, I broached the subject with Rob.

"Do you think we could consider going to see the fireworks? We could leave really early and get a spot before it gets too crowded."

"I think it would be more realistic to host a fireworks show in the backyard than to take Dalia out in a crowd on July 4."

"Okay," I said, taking a deep breath. "Could we maybe go without her?"

It took some convincing, but Rob agreed, so I hired a nurse and a babysitter to stay home with Dalia, and we set out for the fireworks show in a small town nearby.

We found a beautiful spot in a community garden far away from the crowds, where we laid out our blankets and arranged ourselves in a waffle pattern, my head on Rob's lap, Jonah's on mine, and Theo's on Jonah's. It was perfect weather, and as I gazed up at the sky, absently swatting mosquitoes, I thought, *We can do this. We can be great parents to Dalia and still be great parents to Jonah and Theo. We can have moments—whole evenings even—that feel totally normal.* I was peaceful and optimistic and truly happy. The serenity was intense.

It lasted for three minutes.

We had situated ourselves in the wrong spot. We could hear the fireworks, but we couldn't see them over the tree line edging the garden. We craned our necks, spun around, and then, way off in the distance, over the top of the trees, we spotted a few scattered lights.

"Let's go," I yelled, as I shot up and quickly started gathering our blankets in my arms. "If we run to the other side of the field and around those trees, we'll be able to see them!"

We started running, Jonah in the lead. Theo and I were close behind. Rob was bringing up the rear, walking at a leisurely pace.

It was very, very dark. I could barely make out Jonah's shadow up ahead. Theo was clutching my hand, and we ran until we got winded. Theo, who still slept with the hall light on and his door wide open, was getting nervous. "We're almost there," I assured him, trying to sound believable.

"Where's Jonah?" Rob asked when he caught up to us. I'd been so focused on looking down—down at the brambly path and down at Theo—that when I looked up, I realized I couldn't see Jonah ahead. "Jonah!" we called in chorus. "Jonah, where are you?" But all we heard in response were those elusive fireworks.

Before long we heard the crescendo, the unmistakable end to the festivities. Groups of people came toward us carrying folded chairs and blankets, couples walking with their arms around each other, parents balancing sleepy kids on their shoulders.

After five minutes or three hours, Jonah was one of the people walking toward us.

"Hi, Mom," Jonah said casually. "What did you think? Wasn't that cool?"

"What did I think?" I cried, relief spilling out as anger. "I thought you were lost. I thought something happened to you. I thought..."

"Mom, I'm fine. I just wanted to see the show. I thought you were right behind me."

We rode home in complete silence, my mind playing a movie of "worst-case scenario" where Jonah was gone forever.

But he was fine. That was a consolation, even if the rest of us missed the fireworks. Kids get temporarily lost at the supermarket and the park and Disney World all the time. It comes with the territory.

But when we pulled into our driveway, we saw that Dalia's bedroom light was on. It was hours past her bedtime. I raced through the front door and into her room before Rob even turned off the car.

"What's going on?" I asked the nurse, who was standing by Dalia's bed.

"Dalia lost a tooth," she said. "But I'm not quite sure what happened to it."

Rob and the boys came in behind me. "Everything okay?"

"Everything's fine," I said. "Dalia lost a tooth."

"There was a decent amount of blood," the nurse added, "and I used gauze to stop the bleeding, so the tooth might have gotten mixed in with the trash. I'm also wondering if it somehow got flushed down the toilet when she was going to the bathroom before bed."

The five of us—Rob, the boys, the nurse, and I—spent the next twenty minutes picking through the two trash cans in Dalia's room and crawling around the floor with flashlights looking for one of Dalia's tiny baby teeth. Dalia lay dozing in bed the entire time.

The tooth not found, we agreed it must have been flushed down the toilet, as improbable as that seemed. But fifteen minutes later, as Rob and I were getting ready for bed, he suggested we call the pulmonologist.

"Let's just see what he says," Rob said.

"Really?" I turned to him, beyond exhausted and completely done with this night.

"I'm just going to call real quick," he said, the number already dialed.

The doctor listened to Rob's replay of the events. "Yes, I think it makes sense to bring her to the emergency room for an X-ray. We need to be sure the tooth isn't lodged on the trach and doesn't go into her lungs," he explained.

We shouldn't have called. We'd be asleep already if we hadn't.

We didn't even bother getting Dalia dressed. We simply put her in her wheelchair, and she and Rob headed off to the emergency room.

Dalia was rushed in for an X-ray, just minutes after checking in to the hospital.

"Here it is," the technician said to Rob, pointing at his screen.

Rob craned his neck to see the screen without letting go of Dalia's hand and saw that inside Dalia's throat, her baby tooth was sitting on the little internal balloon of the trach we inflated and deflated with a syringe of water multiple times each day. Rob looked from the X-ray to Dalia, who was looking up at him through groggy eyes. "Dad," she mouthed. "My tooth fall out."

After surgery to retrieve the tooth, Dalia was rolled back into her hospital room, sound asleep and clutching a ten-dollar bill. The surgeon moonlit as the tooth fairy.

I went back to work that Monday after the long weekend, relieved to be returning to a job where I felt competent. In my other job, the one that was far more important, the rules kept changing. I tried to give my sons a single normal night, but I failed. I tried to keep my daughter safe, and I couldn't do that without four adults in the house and a whole surgical team at Mass General Hospital.

"How was your Fourth?" people asked by the coffee machine. "Do anything fun?" they asked as we gathered for a meeting. I had two choices. I could tell them the truth: *We tried to go see fireworks and lost our son temporarily. My daughter inhaled her tooth and wound up in the hospital.* Or I could smile with, *It was fine. How about yours?* I didn't want to relive the failed fireworks, didn't have time to explain about the trach itself, let alone the balloon that was inside of it.

I guess we were living in another set of parallel universes too. There was the world at home and the public world we used to fit into with ease. Our life at home felt surreal. Our life outside of home felt like a foreign land where nobody spoke our language. Both felt like the twilight zone.

When I was out in the world without my family, I looked exactly the same as always (give or take ten pounds). But my life had changed so dramatically it shocked me that nobody could tell just by looking at me. Years earlier, when my sister Nomi went out solo for the first time after giving birth to her daughter, Liat, she told me she was surprised every person she interacted with didn't ask her how she felt, how her baby was, what it was like to be a new mom. Her sense of who she was had forever shifted. She wanted the world to keep up.

Now, my sense of self had changed too. There was a chasm between me and the rest of the world, even my most well-meaning friends, because there was no way for me to adequately explain the intensity and fear of my day-to-day existence. Emergency surgery at 2:00 a.m. had to be translated into a visit from an unexpected tooth fairy.

I craved the hours of normalcy when I went to work or spent time with my friends, but I inevitably felt everybody else's life was spinning on a different axis from mine. My home, with the panoply of caregivers and makeshift ICU in Dalia's bedroom, became the one place that made sense to me, even as it kept turning upside down.

28

The Swelling of the Emptiness

Just as we were learning how to live this new life with Dalia, I had to figure out how to live without my father.

A few weeks after Dalia's backyard birthday party, we got a call at midnight from Sharon, my father's best friend.

Rob picked up the phone, and I could hear Sharon wailing through the receiver. "This is horrible," she sobbed. "Leibel is dead."

Leibel, my father, dead? That was impossible.

Sharon must be out of her mind because my father couldn't possibly be dead. Fainted? Maybe. All these years after Nomi died, that was still my go-to explanation. Or maybe my dad had gotten drunk and passed out, which seemed far less believable than him fainting, but much more believable than him dying.

A year earlier, I went to New York for a work event. I was on Weight Watchers at the time and was saving my food points for the fancy dinner, so I didn't eat much during the day. About thirty of us were crowded into a private room at the back of the restaurant, enjoying cocktails and passed appetizers. I had just started sipping my second glass of wine when the woman I was talking to became blurry. I felt a warm flush rise from my toes to my head and started to see black spots. I excused myself, left the private room, walked into the main dining area, and fell to the floor.

Two things were on my mind: one, I am definitely going to die; two, I don't want anyone at the work dinner to know I am dying. When my friend Ilene knelt beside me, I told her both these things. She assured me that one, I wasn't going to die, and two, she'd cover for my absence at the party. Ilene held my arm as I shakily walked to the front of the restaurant, where I called my father.

Fifteen minutes later, my dad came to retrieve me and take me to his New York timeshare, where he miraculously happened to be that night. He made me tea and toast and tucked me in on the sleeper couch. The next morning I was a bit queasy but well enough to go to my meeting.

My dad just needs tea and toast. He just needs Sharon to tuck him in.

I grabbed the phone from Rob. Sharon and I started talking at the same time. "He's dead," she said. "They've been trying to revive him, but he's gone. He collapsed in the elevator after the party."

"Put him on the phone," I said. "Let me talk to him."

"He's gone," she repeated, but still I couldn't believe her.

"Is there an EMT there? Put me on the phone with someone else. I'm sure there's a mistake."

The paramedic got on. "I'm very sorry, miss. We've been working on your father for more than thirty minutes, but we're unable to revive him. We're going to take him to the hospital, where they will officially pronounce him dead." There was no hesitation; no "might be" or "worst-case scenario."

No possibility for tea and toast.

We'd spent the past three months since bringing Dalia home from the hospital in a hypervigilant state. We carefully measured every milliliter of water and liquid nutrition that entered Dalia's body. We monitored her oxygenation and meticulously dosed her medications. All along my father had been by our side; sometimes literally, always figuratively. We were looking so hard in one direction that the blow from the other side was even more shocking.

— ≫ ≪ —

One night, when Rob was on hospital duty and I was at what felt like Jonah's seven hundredth baseball game of the season, I called my dad to wallow. I was so tired, so scared. As I watched Jonah pitch, I talked to my dad on the phone. He listened for a while and tried to cheer me up. Then, thirty-five minutes after we said goodbye, there he was, shuffling onto the sidelines of the field with his walker. He'd left his dinner date and driven the twenty miles to sit by my side.

Another time I called him from Dalia's bedside at the hospital. She was refusing to sleep, and I was frustrated and exhausted. Within an hour, a hospital volunteer wheeled him into the room. My father was tired too. Too tired to walk from the parking lot to the PICU, he found an empty wheelchair and convinced someone to steer him to our room. He pulled up next to the bed and quietly took Dalia's hand. I left the room to use the bathroom down the hall. When I returned, there they were, grandfather and granddaughter hand in hand, both sound asleep.

When I worried one of Dalia's nurses traveling to Africa would come back and infect us with Ebola, my father humored me by researching the precise area she was going to and sending me an article about the precautions being taken in that region.

Now, I was an orphan.

How would I take care of Dalia and be strong for Rob and the boys without my father there to take care of me?

– ›› ‹‹ –

The night after my father died, I was sitting on the lawn in front of my house with two of my friends named Liz. Liz number one, a Harvard PhD, was making a to-do list for me. "I've got the groceries, shiva plans, and house cleaners taken care of," she said. "Do your boys have suits that fit?" Liz number two sat silently, holding my hand.

"It's just too much," I said. "How am I going to get through this?"

Liz number one replied, "You'll get through this. You're a rock."

Liz number two shook her head and said, "It *is* too much. I don't know why any one person should have to deal with so much loss."

They were both right. I'd become a bit of a rock by default. I needed to be shatterproof for my kids. But Liz number two had a point. Hadn't I suffered enough?

I had no illusions that life was fair. I didn't have to look any further than Dalia to see that. And the truth is I'd known for eighteen years that life is a crapshoot, way before Dalia was even born, ever since Nomi dropped dead while playing with her baby. Life wasn't fair. It wasn't fair to Nomi, and it wasn't fair to Dalia.

And yet, shouldn't there be a ceiling on suffering?

I'd never wrestled with the idea of God. My Jewishness was a fundamental part of who I was, much like my family. They were mine, and I accepted them fully, even the bits I found annoying. Whether or not I believed in God didn't make me any more or less Jewish. I believed in God when I said a prayer as my plane took off or when I prayed by mother's side in the hospital.

When Rob and I took the Introduction to Judaism course for his conversion, I was struck by how fully those converting opened themselves up to the nuances of each unit, exploring and debating and questioning the beliefs and traditions we took for granted. I was embarrassed on the occasions when Rob asked, "Why?" and my only answer was "Because."

Now I was angry with the God I didn't even know if I believed in. *Dayeinu*—enough—enough already.

−»‹‹−

My kids' pediatrician called me Job, referring to the biblical prophet who was tested over and over by God. A friend of Rachel's said we were like the Jewish Kennedys, referring not to their looks or money, but to the relentless tragedy that pursued them. My friend Lara, with her inimitable honesty, summed it up like this: "You're so far below rock bottom. You're immersed in molten lava, honey."

The person I really wanted to talk to about my father dying was my father.

I dug out my copy of the book he wrote after Nomi died, *Against the Dying of the Light*. In the book he wrote a letter to Nomi's daughter, Liat, but when I read it that night, I imagined he'd written it for me.

> I think of you, whom I want so much to comfort. I want for you, my love, flesh of my flesh and bone of my bone, that you will be whole. The emptiness cannot be wished away, nor is there reason to try. All we need guard against is the swelling of the emptiness, its displacement of the other truths of our lives.

The emptiness had been there for years by now, growing bigger with each loss.

But there were also beautiful truths that were coming to light. I watched Theo play Candy Land with Dalia, helping her trembling hand move her game piece, and I wondered where his empathy came from. *Why wasn't he acting out, angry that Dalia was taking so much airspace?* I helped Jonah learn to suction Dalia's mouth because, as he put it, "I'm eleven now, Mom; I'm old enough to help." I wasn't surprised when he then said he wanted to be a nurse when he grew up. I saw Dalia's smile, and I wondered how she could find joy while losing almost everything. I watched Rob master the medical minutiae and take care of the tubing and make Dalia laugh with his slapstick humor.

The morning after my father died, I was in bed answering calls. Somehow, between midnight and 9:00 a.m., my world heard the news. Rob had already told the kids. Theo knocked on the door. "Mom? Can I come in?" he said, peeking his head in. He slowly walked over to the bed, balancing a tray with a cup of tea and two pieces of toast. He set them down beside me, crawled into the bed, and snuggled with me. "You need to rest now, Mom," my sweet seven-year-old said. "I made a sign for your door."

"Do Not Disturve. Let Mom Sleep." I still have the sign, and I post it on my door from time to time when I need a few minutes to myself. I reveled in the role reversal, in my chance to be taken care of, if only for a few minutes.

In my dad's book, he wrote, "Sorrow is a truth, but no more than hope; loss is a truth, but no more than love." Sorrow and hope, loss and love were all blossoming within me.

29

In Reverse

Slowly, but not slowly enough, we started moving backward.

I never kept a baby book for any of the three kids, never recorded their first step or word or solid food. Each of their stories started well before I entered the picture, and I knew that any book I could make would be incomplete. I was reminded of how much I'd missed every time I took one of them to a new doctor and later, too, when they started having trouble in school. "When did she roll over?" "When did he start to crawl?" "What was his first word?" *I don't know; I don't know; I don't know.*

But now there was another book taking shape, another I refused to keep. Now, instead of marking major milestones achieved, we tried to ignore the loss of them.

Some of the losses arrived with a swirl of drama—Dalia ate chicken nuggets and potato chips for lunch the day before she was admitted to the hospital in Florida. By the time she was discharged, she'd completely lost her ability to swallow. She never ate again. She spoke her last word right before she was intubated for the final time.

But other losses seeped in, more of a fine mist that settled heavily until the fog was so thick we could hardly see through it.

When Dalia was little, we progressed from diapers to pull-ups to flowered underpants we picked out together at Target. Now she went back to pull-ups. At first, we hitched her underpants right up on top of the pull-up so she wouldn't feel like a baby. After about a year, we didn't bother with the underpants anymore. A couple of years after that, we brought back the diapers. We called them "briefs" rather than "diapers" so she wouldn't feel infantilized. I don't think it made a difference to her at that point, but it did to us.

She'd always been a bit of a fashionista. "She's her mother's daughter," Rob would say as she meticulously chose the perfect dress and leggings and socks for the next day before she went to bed at night. But now she couldn't dress herself. She didn't have the strength or the dexterity. She still had her own sense of style though. I'd pull out three outfit options and hold them up for her to inspect. She'd shake her head no to one after the other. I'd return to the closet and come back with a new selection. She'd reject them all again. I wanted to tell her she had to choose one, that she was being a bit of a prima donna, that we were going to be late.

"She has no say over what's happening to her. This is one of the only things she can control," Rob reminded me, as he brought out three more choices for her to look at. I knew he was right and understood that in my whole body I'd never have as much patience as he had in his pinky.

Once upon a time, when Dalia was able to write, she kept a journal at school in which she recorded the minutiae of her weekend. "I went to get my nails done with Mommy." "I helped Daddy in the yard." "I threw leaves at my brothers."

Once, she surprised me by publishing an entry in her school's Mother's Day cookbook. The theme was "Mom's favorite recipe." Other students submitted recipes for home-made pizza or apple cinnamon buns. According to Dalia, my specialty was chicken nuggets. She wrote, "Ingredients: one package of chicken nuggets, one bottle of ketchup. Directions: go to the store and buy the chicken nuggets and the ketchup and then microwave them at home." The whole town got a copy of the cookbook. I was proud that she'd so perfectly nailed the extent of my culinary skill.

Now, her tremors were too intense to hold the pencil. I'd put my hand over hers to guide her. Sometimes Theo would steer her hand, helping his older sister exactly as she'd helped him when he was learning years earlier. Before long though, her letters were unrecognizable even with a guiding hand. We went back to coloring books, which Dalia could scribble in more easily. We hung the scribbles on the fridge and above her bed.

We had more stuff to carry with us now—special equip-ment and a change of clothes, canned liquid food and all that gauze. It took us more than thirty minutes just to get out of the house. All this was familiar in a way; we'd been through it when each of the kids was little. Back then it was par for the course. We'd share knowing and sympathetic looks with other parents we'd see. Now we were on the receiving end only of the looks—curious, not-knowing stares more often than smiles.

Once in a while we slowed down enough to acknowledge the losses. Rob and I in bed, the overnight nurse watching Dalia, one of us mentioned that the tremors were worse or that Dalia wasn't smiling as much. "I noticed that too," the other would say. Then we'd lapse into silence. Sometimes we held hands or curled into each other. Sometimes we curled away, holding only ourselves.

We tried watching TV as distraction. But there, on what we thought was a comedy, Sandra Bullock used a pen to trach a choking character. They tried it on *Malcolm in the Middle* too. On *How to Get Away with Murder*, somebody said the loss of a child destroys 50 percent of marriages. We curled back into each other.

I knew the very nature of a degenerative disease meant that things would keep changing, that Dalia's illness would progress. And I thought about what that meant. Because my whole life I'd understood progress to mean moving forward, advancing to something better, higher, more refined. But the progression of Dalia's disease was going to do the exact opposite. And not knowing what that would look like—and how we'd all handle it—was the scariest part of all.

30

Present Tense

A few months after my father died, we were officially admitted to the NIH EPI-743 study for an October start date. My immediate reaction was to reach for the phone to call my dad to tell him the news. Sometimes I let myself pretend that he was just on an extended trip to Israel or that his phone was broken. Years earlier I'd practiced what it would feel like when my parents died. Now I tried to remember what it felt like when they were still alive.

To participate in the study, we'd need to go to Washington, DC, for a week every couple of months for at least the next year and a half. Dalia had a fifty-fifty chance of getting the drug instead of a placebo for the first six months. But we were guaranteed that she'd get the actual drug at some point, the drug we knew for a fact her cells had responded to.

"I need to make sure you understand that just because cells respond one way to a drug in a petri dish doesn't mean they'll respond the same way in the human body," the study liaison told us. We didn't need to read between the lines to know she was telling us not to get our hopes up. But we weren't listening. We wanted to get our hopes up.

The whole first week of September I was in daily communication with a cast of characters from NIH—the liaison and the travel coordinator and the research team. We signed dozens of forms. Our travel was booked and paid for, and I explained to my boss that I'd need to be out of the office regularly for trips to DC, though of course I'd work remotely while I was away. I was sent an itinerary, a floor plan of the room we'd stay in, and information about restaurants in the vicinity. It felt like we were embarking on an adventure—like Rob's search for the perfect baby formula in Guatemala times a billion.

The last step was a phone meeting with the nurse practitioner who oversaw the patients once they were admitted to the hospital. I put the call in my work calendar sandwiched between two meetings. It was just a formality in the process, one more step in what had been a five-year journey since Dalia's diagnosis.

"It's Lori Apple, one of the nurse study coordinators. I want to go over logistics with you and make sure we have a full listing of Dalia's medications and daily routines."

I'd prepared for this and pulled out the list of meds I'd printed off the night before. I couldn't pronounce half of them and wasn't sure exactly what each one was for, but I had the names and doses ready. She went over the schedule with me, explaining what each day would look like, when they'd need us for study protocol, and when we'd have free time.

We spoke for about ten minutes before I raised the subject of Dalia's ventilator, which Dalia used 100 percent of the time. "Will Dalia use your ventilator when she's in the hospital, or should we expect her to use her own throughout the visit? I'm just wondering if yours is the same model as ours or if we'll need to learn how to use a different kind of machine."

"Actually, it would be best if she didn't use a ventilator while she's here," Ms. Apple said.

"Well, that's a problem, since she can't breathe without it," I countered, not yet seeing the wall we were about to crash into.

"I'm sorry," she said. "We weren't aware Dalia is ventilator dependent. Is that a new development? Can she go for a few days without it? We really aren't equipped for patients who require ventilators."

The room started to spin. I didn't know what to say. *Rob will know,* I thought. "Can you hold on for a minute while I conference my husband in?"

Rob was more composed than I was. He shifted into medical mode and began explaining the nuances of Dalia's needs, which he'd become far more expert in than I had. He told Ms. Apple how stable Dalia was on the ventilator, that her oxygenation was near perfect and that he and I were fully able to manage that side of things while we were at NIH.

"Please," I begged. "Speak with our doctor. He'll tell you the same thing." She agreed, but her tone said something else entirely: "This isn't going to happen."

My shirt was damp when I hung up the phone. We'd fought bullet ants in a rainforest and swum around great white sharks in the ocean and crossed the Sahara without any water all to reach a mountain we were now being told we weren't allowed to climb.

That night Dalia's pulmonologist called us at home.

"I thought she could do this, I really did," he said. "But after speaking with the team at NIH, I have to agree that Dalia isn't strong enough right now to participate in the study. Even if they could handle her condition when she was there, which is questionable, I don't want her on a commercial airplane."

"We'll drive!" I said.

"Jessie, it's not safe for her to be in the car for that long. Something could happen to the vent or she could be in distress and you'd be stuck. It's just not realistic."

Tears streamed down my face as I grasped for any ray of hope. "What if we break up the car ride into short intervals? What if they ship the drug to you and you administer it?" *What if? What if? What if?*

But it was done. NIH had other kids waiting for Dalia's spot in the study. In fact, they'd probably already called the next child on the list.

We were getting used to loss. We lost the sound of Dalia's sweet voice. We lost our dream of traveling the world with our kids or even driving cross-country. We lost the carefree life we used to have. And now we had to lose the hope that this drug could help Dalia.

I was also losing my belief that if you wanted something desperately enough, if you put all your energy and ingenuity into getting that thing, you could make it happen—a belief that even infertility and Dalia's MERRF diagnosis hadn't burned out of me.

And yet, the whole time I was on the call with the pulmonologist, Rob was putting Dalia to bed. He changed her into pajamas and washed her face and set up her feed. All the while, he was goofing around, helping her smack Theo with her stuffed animal and squirt Jonah with a saline bullet. She was smiling, and the boys were cracking up. "Again," she mouthed, each time they got Jonah wet. After a while, Theo crawled into bed with Dalia, and Rob started reading *Curious George* to them.

Rob wasn't thinking about whether Dalia was in or out of the study or even about the two hours of grading he had left to do later that night. He was entirely consumed by the moment he was in, and this particular moment seemed pretty delightful.

What if I could be more like that? What if I wasn't spending every waking moment thinking about how we could get Dalia better? Could I do that? But if I wasn't trying to fix this situa-tion, who would be? Okay, I bargained with myself, *how about not thinking about it anymore just for tonight? See how that goes, and then decide about tomorrow later.*

If nothing else, it was worth a try.

31

Learning Curve

I tried to keep myself planted firmly in the present, but the ground beneath us kept shifting.

If I let myself breathe for a minute, confident we'd finally put a nursing team together we could count on, someone quit. When we thought Dalia had stabilized, we learned she needed to wear hand braces to slow down the shortening of her ligaments. We got used to those, and then she needed a chest brace so her new spine curvature wouldn't get worse.

And then, just as we were getting in a school routine, we were asked to attend a special meeting "to discuss Dalia's education options."

At this point, Dalia was back at her public school. When she'd returned that fall as a third grader, she could no longer eat or speak or stand. She was attached to a ventilator and had a private nurse in addition to her one-to-one class aide. She stood out before; now you couldn't miss her. But the kids in her class adored her. Isabella sang to her every day during recess. Marcus sent her cards on the days she missed school. Once, when Dalia's nurse called out sick, Rob took the day off work so he could go to school with Dalia.

"How was it?" I asked when he called me at work afterward. "Tell me everything."

"The other kids fought over who got to sit next to Dalia at lunch. They took turns holding her hand whenever we rolled down the hall. So essentially nothing's changed; she's still the center of attention."

But things *had* changed, more than we were prepared to admit. At first, Dalia could go to school for only two hours a day before she became so exhausted she needed to come home to nap. The pace was too rigorous—even in the substantially separate classroom she was now attending. And though the school made all kinds of accommodations for her, she was the exception to every rule. She needed her own special emergency plan for fire drills, her own bathroom, and a private place for the nurse to administer her feedings.

When Rob and I arrived at the meeting, we found eight people seated around the table: the special education coordinator for the district, Dalia's classroom teacher, the school nurse, a guidance counselor, and several others who introduced themselves but whose roles I quickly forgot. They told us that Dalia was the most medically complex child in the entire school district and they simply weren't equipped to meet her needs.

More than seventy thousand people live in this town. How is it possible that Dalia is the most medically complex? How are we winning this contest? Later that night I'd call Rachel. I'd call Cousin Karen. I'd call Lara. I'd tell each of them, "Dalia is the most medically complex child in all of Framingham." I'd say it over and over to see if I could believe it.

"We don't feel we can keep her safe in our public school," said the one who was running the meeting. "We'd like to send her out of district to a specialized school that can meet her needs."

I started to sweat. After all those early years trying to make the case for Dalia to get special services, I instantly found myself arguing the other side.

"She's doing fine with the therapies she's getting," I said. "Her private nurse is able to meet her medical needs, so you don't have to worry about something going wrong at school. She's been through so much change already; please don't make her face even more." *We've gone through so much change already; please don't make us face even more.*

I started scribbling notes to Rob. *Do we have to do this? Are they giving us a choice? What the fuck?* He wrote back: *Let's just hear what they have to say. They can't make us do anything.*

"We'd like you to look at some schools we think would be better for Dalia, and then we can reconvene," someone else jumped in. "We'll make any decisions together, as a team," she added, handing us a list of seven schools and sending us on our way.

I started some perfunctory research, since I knew we weren't going to move Dalia. The first two schools I called cared for children who were developmentally twenty-four months old or younger. The third school wouldn't accommodate a private nurse or a one-to-one aide. *Why did they think these schools would be better for Dalia? Why had any of these been on the list in the first place?*

The seventh school, the Kennedy Day School, was more than an hour away during the morning commute, on the grounds of a hospital. Nobody there was even slightly freaked out by Dalia's ventilator, and when I went to visit, I even met a boy Dalia's age who had a trach. It was clearly the best and only viable option of all the schools on the list, but I hated it anyway.

There were kids with walkers and others in wheelchairs, kids who were totally nonverbal and others who seemed to be making noises they couldn't control. I watched an adult stabilize the hand of a teenage girl to help her write and a ten-year-old boy clasping the hand of an aide as he walked down the hall.

I left in tears. I was crying for the kids I saw, with their gorgeous smiles and broken bodies. I was crying for Dalia, who I feared looked to other parents the way the kids I saw looked to me. I was crying because I couldn't bear to picture Dalia going to school in a hospital. I was crying because I was starting to believe we might not have a choice.

The next day I called the school district representative. "We've gone to visit all the schools on the list, and I have to say none of them makes sense for Dalia. We'd like to keep her in the public school."

"I'm sorry to hear that," she said. "I don't think staying in our school is going to be an option."

That didn't feel very team-like to me. I put on my bravado voice and explained, "I appreciate your position, but we are Dalia's parents and as such we know what's best for her."

"Of course, I understand that, but this is about Dalia's safety. Her needs are too intense for us to handle. There are too many things that could go wrong."

"I'm sure Dalia's safety is more important to me than it is to you. Dalia has a private nurse with her at all times. The nurse's job is to keep her safe, it's not yours—you don't need to worry about that. I'm comfortable with her in the public school, so you need to be okay with this too," I tried.

We could have—and might have—continued like this for hours. Finally, she offered a consultation with an objective mediator to hear both sides and make a recommendation.

I was so tired. I'd been exploring schools and learning about education law and working full-time and taking care of Dalia and trying unsuccessfully to teach Theo to tell time and tending to Jonah's first heartbreak. But I had no time to be tired.

"They're not budging," the mediator told us after we'd lobbed our position back and forth with the school for two days. "If you don't agree, they're going to push for a formal trial with a judge. You'll pay at least $10,000 in legal fees, and it's a virtual certainty you'll lose. You have to understand that most parents go to trial to fight for their children to get special school placements, not to argue against them. No judge is going to overrule a school district that doesn't think it can keep a child safe and feels so strongly about that it's willing to pay tens of thousands of dollars to send that student to a private school to avoid the risk."

"I just can't believe this. I mean, she has medical care with her at all times," I said.

"Jessica, you can send a whole medical team with her to school, but the school system is still liable for her safety. They just can't take that risk."

I didn't want to give in. Part of my job as a marketer for a childcare company was to convey the value of early childhood education. I wrote copy and shot videos and produced ads that told parents choosing a school for their child was one of the most important decisions they'd ever make. Now that choice was being taken away from us.

Can we not even be in charge of where our own daughter goes to school?

"What are we going to do?" I asked Rob as we left the building. He worked in a public school and knew this game better than I did. He was also the one whose emotions were less likely to get in the way. "I don't think we have any choice," he said. "I think Dalia's going to get another thing taken away from her and end up in a place she doesn't belong. I also think we're not going to talk about it anymore tonight, because it's already taken up our whole day."

But the day wasn't over. I called an education lawyer for another opinion. "You'll probably lose," she said. "But at least you'll know you did everything you could."

I called Cousin Karen. "A trial is going to be all-consuming. Is that where you want your energy to be spent for the next several months?"

I leaned back in the rickety Adirondack chair on our front porch. I knew she was right.

"Jess, are you still there?"

"Yeah. I'm here. I'm just thinking about what it's going to look like. I hate this," I said, staring at the old maple tree in our yard, the boys' bikes resting at its feet.

— ❯❯ ❮❮ —

In the fall Dalia entered the equivalent of fourth grade at the Kennedy Day School. The night before she started, I read the daily school schedule and discovered that Dalia would have cooking class on her very first day. How could they make a child who can't eat go to cooking class?

Dalia came home from school that day with a huge smile. The first thing she did was reach into her backpack and pull out four chocolate chip cookies wrapped individually in paper towels. She carefully handed one each to me, Rob, Jonah, and Theo and watched with pride as we ate them and cooed over their deliciousness. When I emailed the teacher to get details on the day, she said the best part by far had been cooking class. "Dalia loved working with the dough, getting her hands gooey and then watching the cookies take shape through the oven door."

When we went to the school a few weeks later to meet with her team, the room was packed with teachers and therapists singing Dalia's praises.

"Dalia is a magnet," said Judi, the classroom teacher. "We all love getting to spend the day with her."

"She's so funny," said Jennifer, the reading specialist. "She demands to read *Judy Moody* every day. She gives us the thumbs-down whenever we pick something that doesn't meet with her approval."

"When I asked her what her favorite color is, she said, 'Sparkles,'" the art teacher added.

The staff got her, and they saw her as a fully realized person.

One after the other, they told us what they adored about her. There, she wasn't the kid with hearing aids, a wheelchair, and a ventilator. She was the kid who went to the Taylor Swift concert and who loved showing off her nail polish and who wore pink and purple clothes every single day.

I realized then that moving Dalia to this school was the best decision we never made.

If she could be so happy about making cookies she couldn't eat, maybe I could choose more happiness too. We started baking at home with Dalia and even got her a chef hat and apron with her name on it.

One day, Dalia and Rob got home from the grocery store, and he wheeled her out of our van onto the driveway. He turned around for a few seconds to put the ramp up and put down the van gate. When he turned back around, Dalia was out in the middle of our lawn, her back to Rob. Her chair had rolled away, spun around, and gained momentum down the small hill at the edge of our lawn. Rob ran to her, terrified, feeling lucky she hadn't tipped over, and certain she'd be scared and furious. He was apologizing through tears before he got to her. When he did, she looked up at him with her huge eyes, smiled, and mouthed, "Do it again!"

Dalia, in spite of everything, was more full of joy than anyone I knew. We started to take her lead and let her happiness be our guidepost.

32

What Can't Be Fixed

It was April, and in true New England fashion, everything was gray—the sky above and the slush below the same shade of melancholy. The day started off like most others: battling with Jonah to get out of bed, trying to convince Theo that a half hour was more than enough time to spend sculpting his hair, forty-five minutes of nursing Dalia before her actual nurse arrived, and a phone call with Rachel on my way into work. She told me she took the day off to get her annual breast MRI and gynecology appointments taken care of. "You have got to be kidding me," I said. "Why didn't you go for the trifecta and get a colonoscopy too?"

Seven hours later, Rachel called me back.

"Rach, this day has been crazy . . . ," I said in lieu of hello. It was all just one ongoing conversation with us, and pleasantries were extraneous. I stopped short because all I could hear was a screaming sobbing on the other end. I'd heard Rachel cry and yell a thousand times. I'd been with her after Nomi died and when each of our parents died too. But I'd never heard this raw, gut-wrenching wailing.

"What's going on?" My legs started shaking, and I reached for the chair behind me.

It took a while, but I was finally able to piece together what she was telling me. Someone from the doctor's office just called to tell her the MRI of her breast showed a large spot on her lung. She needed to go back for tests the next day. When Rachel asked if it might be a smudge on the film, a mistake, a shadow, the doctor replied plainly, "I don't want to give you false hope."

"Rach, there has to be a mistake." I was nervous because it was pouring rain and she was driving, and she was so hysterical. I was way more concerned about her getting into a crash than I was about what the doctor said. It was ludicrous to think that Rachel, who felt perfectly fine, had anything dangerous going on in her lung. Maybe the breast people didn't know what the lungs were supposed to look like. Maybe they were looking at the wrong person's films. Worst-case scenario she had pneumonia, which would be a bummer because she was supposed to go to Europe the following week.

Over the next few weeks, after a half-dozen appointments and countless X-rays and a lung biopsy and second and third opinions, we learned that the doctor's instincts had been right. What showed up on the films wasn't a smudge or a misread or any other kind of benign explanation I spent hours trying to convince Rachel—and myself—was likely. What the doctor saw, and probably recognized before she placed that very first call, was stage 4 lung cancer.

And now there was yet another "after" in the befores and afters that punctuated my life, living in one reality before that horrible call and another ever after. I started researching stage 4 lung cancer. Unlike MERRF syndrome, everyone in the world had heard about lung cancer, so the issue wasn't trying to find information, but rather trying to find information I wanted to believe. One search showed the five-year survival rate for stage 4 lung cancer was 1 percent. Another showed it was 4.7 percent. I searched and searched, trying to find better results, higher percentages. And I prayed that Rachel wasn't doing the same thing.

"I'm going to be okay, right?" she asked me most nights. And I promised her she would be. "There's so much money being funneled into research; we just need to keep you all right until they come up with a cure," I'd say sometimes, suddenly an authority in prognoses. "We can't believe the statistics," I'd try other times. "They include old people and really sick people. Cancer aside, you're young and healthy. You'll beat the odds."

If neither of those approaches worked to ease her fear, I told her we were going to travel the world to find an exotic cure. "We'll go to the rainforests of Cambodia if we need to," I said, having no idea if there were rainforests in Cambodia and, if so, why they might be harboring a cure for cancer.

It was just the two of us left from our family of origin, and we decided together that she'd live until a cure was discovered, if for no other reason than surely God wouldn't take her from me too.

I'm not sure why we were so certain that was where God would draw the line. Never mind the Syrian refugees or the starving Ethiopians or the mass shootings in our own country or the myriad ways people suffer and die all over the world every single day. We were firm in our belief that Rachel would be okay because, as she put it, "God would never do that to you, Jess."

But what about what God had done to her? And what about what God had done to Dalia or to Nomi? I didn't want to examine our logic too closely, because I knew we were entering the realm of magical thinking. We both had to have known we were kidding ourselves, but the idea that God would draw the line here reeled us in when we began to dance too close to the fear.

And besides, there were things to be done. With Dalia, we were helpless if not hopeless. With Rachel, there were so many drug trials and treatment options and specialists to choose from. Together, we chose a hospital and a doctor and a chemo protocol and became experts in yet another illness. There was even a whole floor in the hospital dedicated just to lung disease.

On the first visit to the hospital, we met with a cancer social worker, who gave Rachel a brochure, a map of the neighborhood, and a schedule of classes she could take alongside her treatment, things like yoga and meditation and expressive arts.

"Do I get a mug and a T-shirt too?" Rachel joked. The social worker didn't think that was funny, but I did.

We went to see the cancer nutritionist to learn what foods she should add to her diet and which she should take away.

"What about wine?" Rachel asked.

"You can have a glass of wine now and then," the nutritionist answered.

"So, if I have a glass *now*, can I have one *then* an hour from now?" Rachel asked. The nutritionist didn't think that was funny, but I did.

When Rachel came to me in her darkest moments, my go-to was to try to assuage her fears. I wanted to make her feel better. I told her we were going to celebrate her eightieth birthday and look back on this as a really shitty chapter in the long story of her life.

Sometimes that worked for her. But other times what she needed was for me to just be with her in the anguish. "Jess, please don't try to solve this," she said. But if I couldn't raise her spirits, what value was I offering? I didn't want to cry with her, didn't want her to see my fear in case it compounded hers. But what I wanted or didn't want was irrelevant. When she needed me to hold her in her sorrow, I needed to do that. Later, alone or with Rob, there would be time and space for my own tears.

What I didn't know then was that she might have welcomed my tears. I didn't take what Jonah taught me about loosening my armor and show Rachel that her fears were my fears too. I wish I'd validated her anguish. Instead, we each stayed guarded, trying to protect ourselves and each other from the terror we felt.

I was still most comfortable in problem-solving mode. And there were lots of problems to solve. That was something real I could give her. When she drove to Boston for the chemo appointment but was too wiped out to drive home, I could find her a ride and figure out how to get her car back to her house in New Hampshire. When she needed someone to spend the night with her or check in during the day, I could find a nursing service to fill the gaps. When she ran out of the few foods that didn't make her feel nauseous, I could stock her fridge. But in the end, the real problem—the only one that mattered—would prove too big to be solved.

33

Tunnel Vision

I didn't know if I should keep my eyes open or shut. Open, I could see nothing but darkness. It was pitch black, like the darkness of the Bar Kochba Caves where Rob and I went spelunking in Israel. I loved that adventure for two reasons: first, because it gave me the opportunity to use the word "spelunking"; second, because exploring caves freaked out Rob and didn't scare me at all. In pretty much any other circumstance, I was the one to get nervous, and Rob was the one to calm me down. Turbulence, roller coasters, driving in stormy weather, horror movies, cooking raw chicken—all these made my hands sweat. But put me in a cave and I became Lara Croft.

But now, there was more than just the pervasive darkness to contend with. With my eyes open I could sense the metal tube that contained me, even if I couldn't see it. There was no way to move my hands or sit up. *Shut is better,* I thought. *With my eyes shut I can pretend I'm somewhere else, visualize a beach or a beautiful garden, practice my deep breathing.*

The day had started off uneventfully. It was Columbus Day, so we all had the day off—no school, no work, and no nurses. Rob slept in, and I took care of Dalia's morning routine. Around ten or so, I was out doing some errands when I glanced in the rearview mirror. For some reason, the rearview mirror always exposed things I didn't see elsewhere—the rogue chin hair or the eyeliner smudge. But this time, what I saw was that one of my pupils was dilated, so much so that barely any of my green iris was visible. The other eye looked perfectly normal.

I turned the car around and drove straight home. "Rob, do you see this?" I asked as I ran inside. I put my face a couple of inches away from his and opened my eyes as wide as possible.

"Hmmmm," he paused. "What's going on with your eye?"

"I don't know!" I shouted. "Should I call the doctor?" I asked while googling "one eye dilated."

> Significant size differences or symptoms that come on suddenly can be a sign of dangerous health problems, including a brain aneurysm.

My eyes felt fine, but now I felt like I was going to throw up. "Sweetyheart, why don't you take a picture and send it to David?" It was a great idea. David was a doctor, a brilliant diagnostician, and one of the least alarmist people I knew. So when David said, "Jess, if it doesn't get better by tomorrow, you should probably see your doctor," I knew I had to get it looked at immediately.

Fifteen minutes later, I walked into a drop-in healthcare center.

"I know this is probably ridiculous," I began when the doctor came into the exam room. "But one of my eyes is dilated, and I just figured I should get it checked out."

I was somewhat apologetic, worried the doctor would think I was wasting her time.

"Let me take a look," she said, walking toward me with a smile. But when she saw my eye, her smile disappeared. "I can't evaluate you for this. This could be very serious. You need to go to the emergency room right now."

This could be very serious? What does that mean? Is it a brain aneurysm? A stroke? Now I didn't just feel like I was going to throw up, I felt like I might pass out too.

"I'm sure it's nothing. But if it is something, we both have it, because my left eye was weirdly dilated a few months ago," Rob said, when I called him on my way to the emergency room.

And I remembered the same thing *did* happen to him a few months ago. It resolved within a day, and we chalked it up to a scratched contact lens or the possibility he got chlorine in his eye in the gym pool. It turned out to be nothing, but that didn't assuage my fear now. His voice didn't have the same magical effect it did when he talked me through a snowy winter commute or a bumpy plane ride.

I replayed this conversation as I lay in the MRI machine, the relaxing images I sought of beaches and gardens nowhere to be found.

I wanted to believe the reason I wasn't worried when Rob's eye was dilated was because he wasn't worried, and I took my cues from him. But now I couldn't help but wonder whether the reason I didn't fall apart was because his dilated eye was *his.*

I'd become expert at being strong for other people. I could snuggle next to Rachel in her hospital cot and play word games with her to take her mind off the chemo dripping into her veins or clean up my mother when she mistakenly removed the steri-strips that were holding her skin together after surgery. I could change Dalia's trach tube for God's sake, which needed to be done perfectly and swiftly to ensure she continued breathing.

But now, at the prospect of what I decided was surely a brain tumor, I was undone. I was scared. I felt alone. The spinning wheel had stopped on me this time; I was certain of it.

And why not? A breast MRI revealed stage 4 lung cancer. Mild to moderate hearing loss was an indicator of an ultra-rare degenerative disease. Of course I thought my dilated eye was catastrophic.

I knew that even though Rob would take care of me through the brain surgery I'd obviously need, it would be my mountain to climb. The strongest Sherpa in the world would lighten the load, but he wouldn't be able to make the ascent for me.

I thought about Dalia's strength, replaying the morning rituals we created for each aspect of her care. There were the silly sound effects I made when I moved her from a horizontal position in her bed to a vertical one to put on her chest brace, the counting before wrapping her feeding tube in a towel to absorb any leak, the way we said the full name of the medicine we put under her tongue every morning: "Atropine sulphate ophthalmic solution USP 1 percent, which means it's a whole lot of water and a teeny bit of medicine."

Holy shit. I gave her the atropine today. If I could have, I would have sat right up in that tube because I suddenly realized I probably got some atropine on my finger and rubbed my eye. We used atropine to reduce Dalia's saliva, but it's also used to dilate pupils during eye exams.

The hammering of the MRI machine pounded on, but I was suddenly floating, detached from my body. It felt like Klonopin with a dash of helium. This time, I was given a pass. It was oddly reassuring to find out that devastating news has an opposite and that I would leave this hospital with nothing more than a story. I wanted to stay in the machine, floating, forever.

When my time in the tube was up, I shared my atropine theory with the doctor.

"Well, that's a new one," he said. He told me everything looked fine and discharged me with strict instructions to do a better job washing my hands after giving Dalia her meds.

I called Rachel on my way home. "Rach, I don't know how you do it," I said. As soon as the words were out of my mouth, I wanted to reel them back in. I never knew what to say when people said that to me.

"You give me too much credit. You'd do exactly the same thing." But I knew she was wrong. I was way better at being the Sherpa than the mountaineer.

Later that night I scrubbed my hands raw after giving Dalia her meds. As I rubbed her forehead—still her favorite—I wondered how scared she was.

Most of the time, I was focused on bringing joy and love to Dalia in whatever ways I could think of. There was a lot of goofing around and music and levity. I took a deep breath and said, "Dal, I see you. I want you to know how brave I think you are. You amaze Daddy and me, and Jonah and Theo. I know you're scared. Me too."

She looked up at me and smiled; that she could still do. Her smile gave me courage, and I also saw a bit of a twinkle, as though she were laughing at me for my foolishness of the day. I turned out the light, and we lay together peacefully, the darkness safely enveloping us.

34

Breath

One Saturday morning, several months into Rachel's diagnosis, I was getting Dalia ready for the day—a ninety-minute routine that included things like pounding on her chest to loosen any gunk in her lungs, and changing gauze around her trach and her G-tube (yep, still the gauze), and pulling meds into syringes, and putting the atropine under her tongue (followed by thoroughly washing my hands), and putting drops in her eyes, and setting up her tube feeding, for starters. I was emptying the can of food into the food pump when Rachel called. I put her on speakerphone because I needed one hand to hold the food bag and the other to pour.

"Jess, it really hurts to breathe this morning," she said. "I'm nauseous and light-headed. I'm short of breath, and I have a million things to do today." I looked at Dalia looking up at me, wondering what exactly was going on with her Auntie Ray. I tried to keep it from the kids as much as possible. I figured there was enough sickness in their lives to contend with already.

"Call the doctor. Let's see if they can put you back on steroids," I said.

But Rachel never wanted to call the doctor. She didn't want to add new meds to her repertoire and, on the flip side, didn't want the doctor to take her off meds she was on that might be making her feel shitty but also might be killing the cancer.

"If I don't feel better, I'll call on Monday. There's nobody there on the weekend, anyway."

"Rachel, page the doctor. This is why they gave you the pager number," I urged.

"I don't want them to think I'm a pain in the ass."

We always thought if the doctors liked us, they'd try harder to cure us.

"This is their job. You're not being a pain in the ass. Call the doctor, and call me right back and let me know what he says."

As soon as we hung up, Cousin Karen called. I didn't even bother saying hello when I answered the phone. "Karen, Rach isn't doing well, and I don't know what to do. She's having trouble breathing and I'm here with Dalia and Rach is all alone. I feel like I need to go there and make sure she's okay, but I can't leave Dalia. I'm really scared. What should I do?"

"Jess, take a breath," Karen urged.

My body tensed. "Please don't tell me to breathe. I'll breathe when Rachel and Dalia can breathe."

Of course, I knew what Karen meant. And I knew that Karen, of all people, would never say anything that wasn't well intended.

I was trying so hard to learn to breathe deeply, to be in the moment, to stay calm in the storm—all the while watching Dalia's and Rachel's lungs fail them, watching their breath being taken slowly away.

As for my breathing, it was intermittent. And it looked so different than it used to. Because in the midst of the chaos and the anguish and the fear, there were moments that were pure joy—moments I'd likely have skimmed right over if not for the pervasive intensity—and that's when I breathed.

I could breathe now when Rachel was feeling relaxed—when she was teaching me how to make cocktails with frothy egg whites because we wanted to celebrate that her latest scan showed the tumor had shrunk.

I breathed when she threw her annual Hanukkah party despite worrying that she'd be too tired, too nauseous to make it through. She was the last one singing next to the piano player that night, wondering why everyone had gone home a mere six hours after the party started.

I breathed when we brought the kids to the skateboard park and raced Dalia up and down the skate ramps in her wheelchair while the boys practiced their ollies.

I breathed when we turned Dalia's wheelchair into a sleigh with glow-in-the-dark lights so she'd have the coolest Halloween costume in town. I'd planned that night meticulously, going to all our neighbors' houses two hours before trick-or-treating to drop off nonedible treats so Dalia could have a whole bag full of treats just like the boys.

I breathed when we tied a kite to the arm of the wheelchair so Dalia could make the kite soar.

I don't think I'd have thought twice about any of these moments that now felt so calming, so lovely, before Dalia got

sick, but now the ordinariness of them made them feel somewhat extraordinary. And there was magic in that.

Breathing was diluting the heaviness with frivolity whenever possible. It was all an intricate dance, and sometimes
I handled it more gracefully than others. But Dalia showed
me that you don't need to be able to stand to have awesome
moves. We still had dance parties in the kitchen to obnoxious
rap music, which I tried to play louder than Alexa was comfortable with. Dalia had more rhythm in the slight movement of
her shoulders than most people have in their fully able bodies.
If she could let loose, I wanted to join her. And if that meant
dancing until I was out of breath from spinning, so be it.

A decade or so earlier, at Dalia's baby-naming ceremony,
Rob had read part of Mary Oliver's poem "The Summer Day."

> I don't know exactly what a prayer is.
> I do know how to pay attention, how to fall down
> into the grass, how to kneel down in the grass,
> how to be idle and blessed, how to stroll through
> the fields,
> which is what I have been doing all day.
> Tell me, what else should I have done?
> Doesn't everything die at last, and too soon?
> Tell me, what is it you plan to do
> with your one wild and precious life?

I liked the ring of it, but I didn't really get it. Rob loved it
though, and he taught poetry for God's sake, so I deferred to
him and happily added it to the program.

Now, all these years later, I felt like the poem had been written just for me. I still wasn't able to be idle, but after all this time, I was starting to pay attention.

PART FOUR

Star Light, Star Bright

35

What She Can Do

In our synagogue, dates for bar and bat mitzvah ceremonies are assigned years in advance, way before your child has stopped squirming in the pews or surreptitiously putting their iPad inside the prayer book during services. You know the exact date your child will become an adult—at least in the eyes of the Jewish world—while they're just getting braces and mastering math facts.

We'd known Dalia's bat mitzvah date for years, but now that the date was approaching, we were more than a little ambivalent.

There were practical concerns, of course. Dalia could no longer speak or read, both crucial skills to saying a blessing over and chanting from the Torah. We also had to consider her extreme fatigue. A two-hour service followed by an even longer party would definitely result in a major energy crash.

But then we remembered how worried we were years before when planning Jonah's bar mitzvah. We'd figured Dalia would be exhausted and had hired a nurse and an aide to take her home early. As it crept toward the agreed-upon time of her exit, Rob and I watched Dalia in the center of the dance floor. There she was, beaming from her chair, holding the hands of family members and friends who'd crowded around her, each waiting for a turn to spin and twirl with our seated beauty, who was radiating so much joy. We gave the nurse and the aide the rest of the night off and went to join Dalia on the dance floor. I might have felt a little bad for Jonah, since Dalia was clearly the center of attention and it was, after all, his event, but he was too busy trying to sneak a kiss from Eliana in the photo booth to notice.

How could we take another chance for so much happiness away from our daughter? And, for that matter, we didn't want to deprive her of the opportunity she so deserved, the chance to take her rightful place in our community. Dalia would never learn Hebrew, never go to overnight camp or sing Jewish songs or learn even a single Israeli dance. Yet every time we went to services, Dalia insisted we sit in the front row so she could hear the music clearly, clap her hands, and let loose with her shoulder dance. Her quiet participation in the music emanating from the bimah (the podium at the front of the room) could rival the loudest gospel choir.

There was also what it meant to me. I could still sing my own bat mitzvah portion by heart. I remembered that when my friend Dana's mother saw me shaking before my own service, she did some deep-breathing exercises with me to calm me down. I still had the bracelet my mother gave me and the tiny prayer book gifted to me by the synagogue. Dalia's childhood looked nothing like mine. I wanted one day of overlap. And I wanted the cocktail of nostalgia and pride I'd consumed at Jonah's bar mitzvah.

On top of all that, there was the matter of our boys. Depriving Dalia of a bat mitzvah would have sent them a loud message that Dalia wasn't equipped for or deserving of the same rites of passage they were entitled to. It would be yet another reminder of her difference, rather than a reassurance of her more important sameness.

We scheduled a meeting with a member of the synagogue clergy, Cantor Hollis, to help us think through if—and how—to give Dalia a bat mitzvah. Cantor Hollis is one of those people who always makes you feel a little bit better about yourself and about the world for having someone like her in it. When she sings, you understand that if you believed in angels and if you thought those angels were in the business of singing, this is what their voices would sound like.

"What should we do?" I asked her. "How can Dalia have a bat mitzvah when she can't read or speak and might not even be able to understand what's going on?" We didn't want to make her a spectacle in any way.

"I hear you," Cantor Hollis began. "Let's think about what Dalia *can* do as our starting point, rather than focusing on what she can't."

Dalia couldn't chant Torah, but she could push a button on an iPad. Cantor Hollis told us about a program called Gateways that provides Jewish education to kids with all kinds of abilities. We signed up, and every Sunday Dalia and I spent the morning in a small classroom with other young teens, some in wheelchairs and diapers, some who were silent like Dalia, some who could speak, and others who verbalized in their own unique way. The kids had varying cognitive and physical abilities, but they had one thing in common: every one of them was preparing for an upcoming bar or bat mitzvah ceremony.

The teacher, a woman named Rebecca, sat with Dalia week after week and sang the prayers to her. And on the day of Dalia's bat mitzvah, when Dalia pushed the button on her iPad in time for each prayer and reading of a Torah passage, it would be Rebecca's voice that rang out through the sanctuary.

And that wasn't all. Dalia couldn't write a commentary on the weekly Torah reading, but she could sit with Rob as he wrote one, and she could hold his hand while he read it to the congregation.

Dalia couldn't carry the Torah around the perimeter of the synagogue, but Jonah could, and Theo could push Dalia in her wheelchair beside Jonah as he did so.

And there was the most important thing Dalia *could* do: she was more than capable of celebrating, of joyously being seen as a full member of her community.

Once we decided to throw ourselves into preparing for the bat mitzvah, there was no way I was going to miss the opportunity to make it the most gloriously magical thing Dalia had ever experienced. The decorative motif was obvious—we'd transform the blank canvas of a party room into a bursting field of dahlia flowers. I worked with my friend Susan to envision an obscene abundance of pink and purple dahlias made of construction paper and measured to the exact height of Dalia's sightline from her wheelchair. A little bit Oz-like, maybe a bit Dr. Seuss-esque, but utterly Dalia too.

The most important thing, Cantor Hollis told us, is that we find a way to meet Dalia where she was, so she could have a bat mitzvah that was meaningful to her and honored who she is. And so that's what we prepared to do. We learned yet again that honoring what Dalia could do was worlds more important than grieving what she couldn't. One day, more than likely, there'd be time for that grieving. But that time wasn't now, and we weren't going to waste a minute of her life grieving prematurely.

36

Corners of Beauty

On the eve of my bat mitzvah, my father gave me a letter he had written for the occasion.

> Sweet Jessie, my eternal beloved,
>
> Tomorrow you will become a bat mitzvah. With this rite of passage, it's time for you to fully accept your birthright. You were born into a life of privilege. The privilege is that you come from a tradition of carers. You are *rachmanot bat rachmanim*, the child of compassionate parents and grandparents, and back through the generations. Seek to be a link in that chain, to become, in your turn, the compassionate parent of compassionate children. Make a difference; seek to engage in *tikkun olam*, in repairing the world, in whatever ways are given you, in whatever ways you can.

It was heavy stuff for a not-yet-thirteen-year-old, but I sensed, even then, that I should tuck it for safekeeping in the box marked "super secret" on the top shelf of my closet, in between my pleather diaries with the little silver locks and keys.

This was the context in which I learned what the expectations were for who I would become. At the time, I was far more focused on whether Luke and Laura would end up together on *General Hospital* and on reliving my first kiss—forty-two seconds with Steve Gerden in the middle of Foster Field—than on thinking about things like repairing the world.

It would be many decades before I read that letter again. My super-secret box had moved from my childhood house in Brookline to the basement of Nomi's house, where I trusted her to keep it safe. Rob and I were living in our small apartment then. There was no room for extra boxes, and besides, I didn't think having a box labeled "super secret" would be a great way to kick off our life together. By the time Nomi died, I'd forgotten about the box altogether, until the night my brother-in-law David called to tell me his basement flooded. In weeding through the destroyed electronics and dripping piles of books, he came across a drenched box with my name on it. "Everything was destroyed. I tossed it all," he said.

Fast-forward about twenty years. Rachel's cancer was blossoming. On Thanksgiving, she came over to our house with two things: a huge stuffed Rainbow Dash for Dalia that was almost as big as Dalia herself, and a sealed envelope with my name on it in my father's signature all-caps handwriting.

"I've been going through boxes of Dad's stuff," she told me, handing me the envelope. "This is yours."

"Oh my God, Rach. What is this?"

She glanced up while leaning over to kiss Dalia.

"I have no idea. Do you have any appetizers put out yet?"

"Wait," I said, handing her some cashews. "Is there any piece of us that thinks this could be money?"

"If it is, we're splitting it 50/50."

I started reading aloud.

> Sweet Jessie, my eternal beloved,
> Tomorrow you will become a bat mitzvah.

The words were familiar. It was the very letter he'd written to me all those years ago. My dad loved his own writing and apparently kept a copy of the letter for himself.

But the next bit, after the instruction to repair the world, was unfamiliar. If it was in the original, I had forgotten it completely.

> Be gentle, always. The world is so raucous, there is so very much noise. Do not add to that noise. Instead, create a corner of quiet, of peace, and of grace. There are, every day, corners of beauty, and one day there will be a world of beauty. Our task is to encourage that world. This is not a burden, not at all; but a way of life, a perspective. These are not the words of a sermon, but of a father who loves you and wants the best for you, wants your happiness, and knows whence you come, hence where you are intended to go.

The hair on my arms stood at full attention. It was a message from my father from the grave.

Encouraging a world of beauty seemed like an assignment that was way out of my reach. It's not that I didn't care about the forest anymore, it was just that my own trees took every bit of energy I had. But corners of beauty? That was a concept I could get behind. Because even though my life had been sadder and scarier than my dad could have imagined when he wrote those words, it turns out Rob and I had been creating corners of beauty all along, carving out space for joy and laughter in what might have been a life overcome by darkness and fear.

— ❯❯ ❮❮ —

A lifetime earlier, at my college graduation, Nomi gave me a framed poster she'd made for the occasion. My sisters and I were never into arts and crafts. We didn't draw well or know how to sew or knit or paint. So the fact that Nomi made a poster for me would have been meaningful no matter what was on it. But the words she carefully wrote inside a mosaic of colored boxes she had drawn imprinted on me.

The poem was part of "Desiderata," written by Max Ehrmann in 1927.

> You are a child of the universe no less than the trees and the stars; you have a right to be here.

> And whether or not it is clear to you, no doubt the universe is unfolding as it should. Therefore be at peace with God, whatever you conceive God to be.

> With all its noise, sham, drudgery, and bro-
> ken dreams, it is still a beautiful world. Strive
> to be happy.

My father's letter spoke about creating a world of beauty. Nomi's poster recognized that within the chaos and disappointment, it was already a beautiful world. My dad asked me to take responsibility for making things better, where Nomi reminded me to appreciate what was already there. Neither was given to me at a time in my life when I was ready to accept the charge.

But through Dalia, and Rob and Jonah and Theo, too, I was now learning to do what both my father and Nomi asked of me. The fact that neither my father nor Nomi was there to cheer me on pierced me. But I also felt that maybe, if they had any inkling of how things were playing out—not of how my dreams were broken, but of how they were being entirely reshaped—they'd be proud of me.

37

Light Up the Tunnel

The last time I wore a headlamp was twenty-five years ago when I went camping to impress Rob. We slept in a tent on the side of a mountain we'd spent the better part of the day climbing. It was romantic and adventurous and sporty, but it was cold and uncomfortable and tiring too. Once he became my husband, I decided I didn't have to go camping anymore.

Then, I wore the headlamp hopefully. This time, I wore it desperately, since it was the only way I could see the small, portable generator I was filling with gas in our driveway. It was freezing outside, but it was freezing inside the house too. I looked at the diagram Rob drew for me so I'd know where to put the gas and how to start the generator back up, having studied the warnings and convinced myself that a simple mistake might start a fire or get me electrocuted . . . or both. And the longer I stayed outside trying to make sense of the directions, the more I began to worry about frostbite too.

We'd been without electricity for two and a half days thanks to a windstorm that knocked out the power lines. For our neighbors it was an inconvenience, no light or heat or hot water. For us, it was something else entirely. We didn't just need electricity for comfort; we needed it to run the equipment Dalia depended on to stay alive. We ran one hundred feet or so of extension cord through the garage and across the house into Dalia's room, so we could plug in her ventilator, her food pump, and a small space heater.

Incidental to the gravity of the situation was the fact that Dalia's bat mitzvah was in two days. We'd be hosting 150 people at the synagogue, which would be followed by a party that resembles a wedding, without the groom. Later that night, when the machines were humming as they're supposed to, I'd put on two sweaters and a down puffer coat, set myself up at the kitchen table, and use the headlamp to illuminate the seating charts I'd yet to finalize.

The year before, I helped Rachel plan her son Jake's bar mitzvah, which she unapologetically referred to as "her" bar mitzvah—the irony of course being that she was neither thirteen nor a boy. I helped her obsess over playlists and menu options and dress selections, and I worried alongside her about whether Jake would master his Torah reading, which is central to the entire proposition. We knew Dalia's bat mitzvah would resemble that more traditional event in name only, and we imagined all kinds of "what ifs" leading up to the big day. But needing to find a workaround for the electricity that kept her alive hadn't made our list.

Rob was inside getting Dalia out of bed after her nap. Thirteen years old, she weighed nearly a hundred pounds, and the safest way to transfer her from the bed to her wheelchair was with a ceiling lift, an upgrade from the utilitarian lift delivered to the house years before. But the lift, too, needed electricity to run. I was promoted (or maybe demoted, I'm not really sure) to generator duty while Rob moved Dalia. Jonah and Theo and Shawna were huddled in Dalia's room, since that's where the action was, and also because it was the warmest room in the house.

My life is a shit show, I thought to myself for the seventeenth time that day as I turned the generator valve and moved the thing that apparently is called the choke and flipped the switch to the "on" position and pulled the cord. And then, lo and behold, I heard the generator kick on.

"It's working!" I heard Rob call from inside as I dashed into the house to escape the freezing rain. I moved through the darkness of the living room and kitchen. And then, as I made my way down the hall, I saw a warm glow emanating from Dalia's bedroom. I entered to find that her room had been transformed. Shawna and the boys had strung the battery-operated twinkly white lights I bought for Thanksgiving around the room. There were other lights too. Lanterns from the party we threw last summer sat on the bookshelf, and lit candles outshone the glowing numbers on Dalia's oximeter and ventilator.

They took the clip-on, battery-operated reading light we purchased earlier that day at CVS and put it on one of the arms of Dalia's wheelchair. Rob was ensuring all the medical equipment was working as it should, while Shawna tried to scare the kids with ghost stories.

And for a moment or two, I was in the scene but also outside of it. It was terrifying, not just because of the power outage, because that day it was a power outage and the day before it was a high fever and tomorrow it would be something else we couldn't yet begin to imagine. We were always on the precipice, one small step away from tragedy.

But we'd made our own little corner of beauty too. There were the kids, who by some stroke of luck or twist of fate came to us all those years ago from a country thousands of miles away. There was Shawna, who walked into our house for a temp job and, for reasons I couldn't fathom but for which I was eternally grateful, never left. And there was Rob, whose steadfastness made the whole operation run smoothly, and who didn't ask me to go camping anymore. And there were those twinkly lights, which can make even a power outage seem celebratory.

And I was reminded that somewhere in the darkness there's always light to be found.

"Who wants to play hide-and-go-seek?" Shawna asked, as she started running into the blackness beyond Dalia's room.

"You're it!" Theo shrieked, bolting out in front of her.

"Ready or not, here we come!" I said, pushing Dalia's chair, her light leading our way.

38

Twirling Together

One night I crawled into bed next to Rob, who was already there reading. We never actually got into bed at the same time, since one of us stayed in Dalia's room until the overnight nurse arrived. I was "it" on this night, and now I was both wired and bleary-eyed, worried I was too tired to fall asleep, which seemed like a cruel irony.

Rob was in the middle of teaching the tragedy unit of his sophomore literature course and was rereading James Baldwin's essay "The Uses of the Blues." I curled up next to him.

"Can we watch an episode?" I asked, wanting to keep going with *The Sinner* on Netflix.

"I have to finish this first," he said, knowing, as I did, that I'd be asleep within minutes if we turned on the TV.

I snuggled in a bit deeper, looked up from his chest, and glanced at the underlined bits in the book he was holding. Baldwin wrote that even when things are a complete mess and there's nothing you can do about it, you still have do something about it.

Holy shit! Yes, James Baldwin, it *is* a mess, and no, I can't do anything about it. I had just taped Dalia's eyes closed, which I now had to do at night, since she had lost the ability to blink and her corneas were drying out. My soundtrack at the time was the simultaneously heartbreaking and reassuring rhythmic hissing of her ventilator.

I grabbed the book out of Rob's hands and read more. Baldwin was writing about the struggles of Bessie Smith, a blues singer whose life couldn't be more different from mine. He was writing about not giving up, not looking back in the face of tragedy and trauma. What did Bessie do instead? According to her song "Long Old Road," she picked up her bag and carried on.

And there, in the words of a black civil rights activist, I saw myself. And in that seeing I felt less alone.

I suddenly remembered why classics were classics, and why universal ideas were universal, and why there was such a fuss made over James Baldwin. He knew what he was talking about.

Yes, my life was a mess, and I couldn't do anything about it. I couldn't wish away Dalia's disease. I couldn't get her into a research study that would miraculously cure her. I couldn't slow the degeneration or come up with an adequate answer when she and the boys asked why this, any of this, had to happen. And I couldn't get pregnant or make my mother eat or grow old with my sisters.

Baldwin wrote that even amid the mess, you have to do something about it.

So, what did I do? For one thing, I had awesome girls' days with Dalia. They didn't look like what I said I wanted that night when Rob and I were on our dinner date years before.

They were much harder, that's for sure. But they were also more special. Dalia loved getting her hair and nails done. We found a place that could accommodate her wheelchair and ventilator and where the nail technicians didn't mind that our appointment took twice as long as anyone else's, since we had to stop periodically for me to suction Dalia. Her tremors made her hands shake, so I steadied her palms from underneath while her nails were painted. She always picked pink and purple, not wanting to choose between her two favorites.

Somewhere along the way, we all decided that we wouldn't stop doing things just because they were hard. We ate at restaurants even though Rob had to prop Dalia up with one of his arms for the entire meal so she didn't slide down in the booth. We found a beach that had an access mat on top of the sand so we could roll Dalia onto the dock, pink fishing rod in hand. And everywhere, always, we tried to ignore the stares. That may have been the hardest part of all, especially for the boys. I wanted to be gracious, to appreciate that most people had probably never seen a person with a tube coming out of her neck before. But I couldn't always summon the grace. Sometimes I opened my eyes as wide as possible and stared right back until the person looked away.

I don't know how much of the refusal to yield to the struggle the kids learned from us and how much we learned from them. Once, when Theo and I were holding Dalia's hands on our way into their childcare center, he turned to me and said, "We show the trouble who's boss, right, Mom?" Was this, too, from *Wonder Pets*? I didn't know, but it became part of my mantra.

And sweet Dalia, by the time of her bat mitzvah, couldn't speak. She couldn't eat. She had only periodic and limited control of her arms and legs, which most people consider essentials for dancing. But none of that stopped Dalia.

If dancing is a celebration of life, a warding off of tragedy, a reminder of just how much living there is yet to come, then as Dalia danced that night—needing help to move her arms to the music, needing to be guided in and out of the hora lines, hand in hand, spinning inside the circle of dancing family and friends—she drove her tragedy not just into a corner, but out of the synagogue and into the night as well.

What it took James Baldwin twenty pages to articulate, and what it had taken Rob and me more than a decade to figure out, Dalia knew intuitively and put on display from a wheelchair, without even the benefit of her voice: tragedy may be powerful, but I'm much, much stronger.

And I'm a lot more fun at a party.

We were worlds away from a jazz club in Harlem, and the songs of the hora sounded about as different from the blues as you can get. But the triumph in our music, in our dancing, in the love that showered Dalia that day, was the five of us coming together to transcend the suffering.

We didn't know what Dalia's future would look like, and we could spend each day frantically consumed by the fear and uncertainty. But if we did, we'd be wasting the present.

I didn't want to miss a minute of dancing with Dalia. I knew that the dance would always include losses—those that had already happened and those that were yet to come—but I'd lose so much more by sitting those dances out. We spun on the dance floor, and I looked up at the high ceiling of the synagogue, realizing that this was what life felt like, the joy and the sorrow weaving in and out—sometimes taking turns, sometimes twirling together, each more powerful because of the other.

— ❯❯ ❮❮ —

Once upon a time this is how the story ended. Here, in a moment in a day in a place where joy was much louder than sorrow.

They were both there, of course. By then we knew that sorrow wasn't going away. But we also knew they could exist together. Sorrow was growing, and there were times when its big shoulders pushed joy into a tiny corner. But joy was stubborn. Dalia took Blackie-O for a spin on her wheelchair or Rob brought a new Amelia Bedelia book home or we threw an "it's nobody's birthday party," and joy came dancing back to center stage. And so it was.

But there's more to the story.

Epilogue

Four years and one day after her bat mitzvah, Dalia died.

Ever so slowly, but also in a single minute, the disease took over. Dalia's facial muscles weakened, and she couldn't mouth words anymore. Her fingers became too shaky for her to use her communication device and then even too shaky for her to point to what she wanted. More time passed and she wasn't able to nod yes or shake her head no. And then she couldn't move at all. She couldn't even blink. It seemed, at times, as though she were disappearing, fading backward into the disease she'd never let define her.

I kind of wished I'd known the last time she smiled that it would be her last. I would have fixed my attention so powerfully that the memory would have imprinted in every crevice of my brain. But I was also glad I hadn't known. I might have stopped smiling too.

The pandemic came, and suddenly we were home all the time. The parade of people in and out of our house thinned. It was the five of us and Blackie-O. Nurse Jane, Nurse Lori, and Nurse Grace took turns caring for Dalia, but half our nursing shifts went unfilled. Like everyone, we hunkered down. And in some ways the hunkering was a blessing. We didn't have to waste time doing anything but being together.

We could see the disease's impact on Dalia's body, but there was no way to know how much the disease had spread its tentacles through her brain. We treated her as though she could understand everything that was happening. We talked to her constantly; got her out of bed, dressed, and into her chair; brought her wherever we were in the house; went outside for long walks. But I also prayed she wasn't aware of what was happening. I wanted to believe she was in more of a dreamy peaceful state than aware of the nightmare.

Then one day Dalia's neurologist called to tell us she was enrolling for a new EPI-743 clinical trial right here in Boston. The drug had a new name now, but it was the same one I'd worked so hard to get her access to years earlier. Dalia was in if we wanted her to be. In fact, she'd be the first person enrolled in Boston. "It isn't going to change the trajectory for Dalia," the doctor said. "But she'll help us learn and possibly make a difference for children in the future."

We decided to go for it. The idea of Dalia helping even one other person with this insidious disease was powerful. And the sliver of hope it gave us was even more powerful. The doctors could tell us it wouldn't change the course for Dalia, but what if they were underestimating? What if this drug turned out to be a miracle? Wasn't the five of us finding each other and becoming a family proof that miracles happen?

So we went back to the hospital for Dalia's body to be poked and prodded. The nurses collected Dalia's urine and drew her blood and measured this thing and that thing while Dalia and I curled together on the hospital bed watching *Encanto*, *Moana*, and *Coco*. After ten hours, we got to go home. Leaving the hospital so quickly felt like a miracle in itself.

We added three more syringes of medicine to the fifteen we already gave her each day. We watched Dalia more carefully to see whether her tremors improved. We were supposed to record how many seizures she had every twenty-four hours, but there were too many to count.

The surface illnesses on top of the disease became more frequent. A relentless stomach bug. An eye infection. A three-week cold. The machines that kept Dalia alive all these years couldn't keep up with the disease progression. We needed to give Dalia a bit of supplemental oxygen. Then we needed to give her a lot of supplemental oxygen. We had to increase the settings on the ventilator to push her lungs harder so she could get more air.

We listened to what Dalia's body was telling us. She was done.

Now the doctors came to Dalia. The neurologist and the pediatrician and the palliative care team. They confirmed what we already knew. "She's near the end," they said.

Dalia's room, the center of gravity for our whole family, was quieter, calmer. We whispered. We replaced the Taylor Swift soundtrack with George Winston. We invited a few of the people who loved Dalia most to come say goodbye.

On the morning of the day, we formed a circle around Dalia's bed. Rob and I were on either side of her, stroking her forehead as we had every single day since the foster mother told us it was Dalia's favorite. Theo was there, of course, as was Jonah, who was now Jojo and well on their way to becoming an EMT. Cousin Karen and Kara and Nurse Jane were there too. There were other people in the room with us: my sisters Rachel and Nomi, my parents, Rob's dad, Dalia's birth mother. We carried them in our hearts, and I knew Dalia was in their circle now.

Cantor Hollis was there. too, singing the same song she'd sung to Dalia sixteen years earlier.

> *L'chi lach* [go forth], to a land that I will show you
> *Leich l'cha*, to a place you do not know
> *L'chi lach*, on your journey I will bless you
> And you shall be a blessing
> And you shall be a blessing
> And you shall be a blessing *l'chi lach*.

And she was.

Dalia was a princess warrior dressed in a sparkly purple gown with a crown of glorious black velvet. She got on her horse every day and went to battle. But her battle wasn't about fighting what was happening to her body. She didn't fight against what wasn't fair or fight for an answer to the questions that had no answer, like "why?"—things she had every reason to rage against. Her mission was altogether different: to embody joy and love despite everything. And that joy and love reflected back to us so we had even more to give her, becoming a virtuous circle.

Even then, at her bedside, in the worst moment of my life, I knew unequivocally that I was blessed to be Dalia's mother. She was born in a different country, in a village I had never heard of, to a woman I couldn't speak to without an inter-preter, and we'd been intertwined at an adoption agency in an office park in a Boston suburb.

Who would I be now if just one thing had been different? Rob and I could have gotten pregnant. We could have decided to adopt domestically. We could have been matched with a different baby. We could have found out about Dalia's diag-nosis before accepting the match. A thousand circumstances had to align for us to be gifted with our precious little girl. And she was perfect in every way except in the one horrible way she wasn't. How could I not feel blessed?

And if blessed, then perhaps also cursed. This was the paradox I'd been living with for years. There'd been far too much grief—my parents, my sisters, my daughter. But grief is a testament to love. And I'd loved, and been loved, big.

I'd need to decide whether the blessing or the curse defined me. Dalia made that very decision every day of her life in her expansive silent laughter and her magical smile and her uninhibited shoulder dance when her shoulders were all she could move. She made that decision so seamlessly, so grace-fully, as if to suggest it wasn't a choice at all.

Joy and love outshine the darkness and the pain. Dalia knew that intuitively, and I felt I'd get there too. If I needed help, I'd think of Dalia, who could laugh in a world that tried mercilessly to steal her laughter away.

For now, I squeezed Dalia's little hand that would never again squeeze back and just took a breath.

Resources

The people I've met have been my greatest resources along the way. These organizations and books provide education, support, and inspiration.

Gateways for Jewish Education: Access to Jewish Education
(www.jgateways.org):
Providing special education services, expertise, and support to enable students to succeed in Jewish educational settings and participate meaningfully in Jewish life.

Give Kids the World Village
(www.gktw.org):
A storybook resort in Florida where children with critical illnesses and their families are treated to weeklong, cost-free vacations.

Littlewishes.org
(www.littlewishes.org):
Granting the immediate and ongoing wishes of chronically and critically ill hospitalized children to ease their discomfort and bring them moments of joy.

Magic Wheelchair
(www.magicwheelchair.org):
Building epic costumes for children in wheelchairs at no cost to their families.

RECOMMENDED BOOKS

Cervantes, Kelly. *Normal Broken; The Grief Companion for When It's Time to Heal but You're Not Sure You Want To*. Dallas: BenBella Books, 2023.

Devine, Megan. *It's Okay That You're Not Okay: Meeting Grief and Loss in a Culture That Doesn't Understand*. Louisville, CO: Sounds True, 2017.

Didion, Joan. *The Year of Magical Thinking*. New York: Knopf, 2005.

Harris, Dan. *Meditation for Fidgety Skeptics*. New York: Random House, 2017.

Oliver, Mary. *Devotions*. New York: Penguin, 2020.

Rapp Black, Emily. *The Still Point of the Turning World*. New York: Penguin, 2013.

Sarazin, Stephanie. *Soul Broken: A Guidebook for Your Journey through Ambiguous Grief*. New York: Balance, 2022.

Sethi, Tanmeet. *Joy Is My Justice: Reclaim What Is Yours*. New York: Hachette Go, 2023.

Acknowledgments

While this book is intensely personal, it couldn't have come to life without the love, guidance, and support of my village.

I'm tremendously grateful to my agent, Michele Martin, for believing in the book from the start and for being its champion every step of the way. The team at Behrman House: David Behrman, Aviva Gutnick, Dena Neusner, and Vicki Weber, treated the book—and me—with loving care and attention, helping to uncover the essence of my story amid the many hundreds of pages we started with. I'm honored to be part of a publishing family that values its writers and their process as much as it values the product.

Writing a book is only the first step. Getting it into the world is a team sport.

Thank you to the Book Mama herself, Linda Sivertsen, for providing magical time and space in Carmel and for impeccable guidance along the way. Allison Lane is my guru for book-industry ins and outs and her let's-get-it-done approach. Thank you for letting me keep you on speed dial.

I'm indebted to everyone who read versions or parts of the book over the years and offered honest and valuable feedback, including Tamara Dalton, Cheryl Jones, Betsy Rapoport, Caroline Leavitt, and several others.

The doctors, nurses, and caregivers who supported us throughout Dalia's life became an extended part of our family. Their expertise and friendship sustained all of us. I am eternally grateful to our quarterback, Dr. David Landis, doctors Melissa Walker, Patricia O'Malley, and Mary Shannon Fracchia; nurses Jane Scott, Connie Jaroway, Lori Gerulskis, Karen Manning, and Grace Rosa; and the caregivers and teachers who shared their hearts and time with Dalia: Shawna Clark, Kim Meredith, Nicole Pintard, Judi Maggelet, Karla Germain, Stephanie Collier and Melissa Wells.

Meeting other rare parents along the way inspired and helped sustain me. I'm so glad to count these warriors as my friends: Effie Parks, Patti Hall, Daniel DeFabio, Susan Geoghegan, and Nikki McIntosh.

Special thanks to Rosemerry Wahtola Trommer for allowing me to reprint a portion of her poem in the epigraph. Her blog can be found at www.ahundredfallingveils.com. Sign up for her gorgeous daily poems delivered to your inbox.

My sisters of the heart are an essential part of who I am. The newest came onto the scene 25 years ago and the others have been in my life much longer: Dana Snyder, Lara Srinivasan, Kara Dukakis, Jennifer Bailey, Dhana Gilbert, Kim Gouin, Karen Flood, Ilene Serpa, and Terri Queler. Liz Reef is part of this bunch, the boots to my sneakers, a true partner who kept me going and promised me "it was already done" even when I was just beginning.

I am left with a small but mighty family. Liat Deener Chodirker, though you are half my age, you are the person I want to be when I grow up. Karen Fein, you're my cousin, yes, but also a sister and best friend. Sharon Cohen, you are so much more than just my fairy clothes mother. Thank you for staying by my side through it all. My in-laws, Barb and Jim Flaggert, rolled with so much change and were exquisite grandparents to our kids. And Marisol Flaggert, the joy you brought to Dalia makes my heart smile.

My sisters and parents inform so much of what I do. I will keep sharing their stories and talking about them to anyone who will listen.

Ultimately this book is for, about, and of my three children and my husband. Jojo, you made me a mother and continue to teach me about unconditional love. Your resilience and courage inspire me every day. Theo, your smile is magic. If we could bottle your energy and goodness the world would be a better place. Dalia, your light and love continue to guide me.

And Rob. You are my partner, my love, my home, and my heart.

About the Author

Jessica Fein is an author, marketing executive, and a former opinion columnist for the *Boston Globe*. She writes the blog "Grace in Grief" for *Psychology Today* and hosts the podcast *I Don't Know How You Do It*, which features people who triumph over seemingly impossible challenges. Jessica serves on the Board of Directors of MitoAction, an education and advocacy organization for mitochondrial disease. She and her family live outside of Boston.

jessicafeinstories.com

Reading group discussion questions available.